RHEUMATOLOGY

FOR MEDICAL STUDENTS AND JUNIOR DOCTORS

2nd Edition

Dr Matthew Langtree

Department of Rheumatology
Leicester Royal Infirmary
Leicester, UK

Published in the United Kingdom by

Stafford Books
Email: info@staffordbooks.co.uk

First printed August 2011

Second edition printed April 2012

ISBN 978-0-9571563-1-9

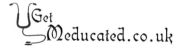

CONTENTS

Dedicated to Laura, Alistair, Olivia and Emelia, without whose love and support this book would not have been possible.

PREFACE

Rheumatology is one of those areas of medicine that often feels slightly neglected. Even though musculoskeletal complaints are extremely common, and the difference a rheumatologist can make to the lives of their patients is immense, it is disappointing that when students or junior doctors rotate to the department, their level of basic rheumatology knowledge is poor, especially when compared to starting in other specialities.

With a standard rheumatology textbook, it very easy to become lost in all the detail and fail to pick up on the key concepts and clinically relevant details. Whilst all that detail is important, sometimes what is needed is a basic, simple and to the point summary of the important conditions. That is what this book aims to provide. As such it is an ideal revision aid for examinations. It can also be used on the ward or in clinic as a quick reference guide. Non specialists and general practitioners should also find that the accessible layout keeps the pertinent clinical information at one's fingertips.

Additionally, I always wished my textbooks had more colour!

Matthew Langtree, July 2011

The author would like to acknowledge Deborah Long, Sarah Parker, Beth Goundry, Laura Bell, Rebecca Neame and Waji Hassan for their helpful comments and suggestions as this book was being produced.

RHEUMATOLOGICAL HISTORY

A good doctor patient consultation is vital in rheumatology. Not only in terms of diagnosis, but for patient satisfaction and therefore compliance with therapy.

BASICS

- Introduction
- Sex
- Age
- Ethnicity
- Handedness
- Occupation

PRESENTING COMPLAINT(S)

- Ask open questions about the presenting complaint(s)
- Ensure you ask about which symptom occurred first, and the order of subsequent symptoms
- Relate these symptoms (and others revealed later) to functional ability

JOINTS

- When asking about joint symptoms, think about how many, which (large, small or both, weight-bearing or non weight-bearing) and symmetry
- Pain – conduct a standard pain history as for any other body area, including timing, especially night pain that wakes the patient from sleep, pain right now, relationship to rest and movement and the effectiveness of any analgesia tried
- Stiffness – when, where and how long does it last until maximal improvement
- Swelling – when, where, relationship to activity and how long does it last
- Deformity – where, for how long and speed of progression

ASSOCIATED SYMPTOMS

- Rashes
- Photosensitivity
- Nodules
- Psoriasis
- Changes in skin pigmentation
- Raynaud's phenomenon
- Alopecia
- Dry or red eyes
- Dry mouth
- Ulcers (oral, nasal or genital)
- Dysphagia
- Dyspnoea
- Loss of sensation or pins and needles
- Myalgia
- Muscle weakness
- Headaches, particularly migraines
- Cognitive disturbance
- Depression
- Seizures
- Fever
- Weight loss
- Change of bowel habit

ADDITIONALLY

- Flares – frequency, severity (did it require hospitalisation), what exactly happened and which joints or parts of the body were affected
- Functional disability – at a minimum ask about cooking (including opening jars), washing, dressing (including buttons and zips), overhead activities, walking distance and ability to climb stairs
- Previous treatments – ask specifically about oral medications, injections, intravenous therapies, physiotherapy and surgery. For each, ask about duration and effectiveness. This not only helps establish severity, but can also inform future treatment options

RHEUMATOLOGICAL HISTORY

PAST MEDICAL HISTORY

- Any condition relating to the presenting complaint
- Psoriasis
- Inflammatory bowel disease or irritable bowel syndrome
- Hypertension
- Gout
- Recurrent infections
- Trauma, including tick bites
- Foetal loss
- Pulmonary embolism or deep vein thrombosis
- Blood transfusions or tattoos
- Travel history
- Sexually transmitted infections
- Any significant cardiorespiratory condition
- Any significant gastrointestinal or genitourinary condition
- Medication history, including over the counter and illicit drugs
- Allergies

- Ask an open question about family history, but then specifically ask about arthritis (any type and note the age of onset), inflammatory bowel disease, psoriasis, gout, Marfan syndrome, Ehlers-Danlos syndrome and ankylosing spondylitis
- Enquire about home circumstances, including type of property (and floor if a flat), co-inhabitants and relationship, stairs including outdoor steps and any adaptations already made
- Ask about smoking history, alcohol intake (past and present), recent stressful events, ability to relax or sleep and sexual history

ADDITIONAL POINTERS

- Establish whether symptoms are acute or chronic
- Pain – inflammatory pain often presents at or after rest, whereas non-inflammatory pain is more directly related to use. Severe bone pain is classically unremitting and persists throughout the night, disturbing sleep
- Stiffness – when related to osteoarthritis tends to last for less than 30 minutes after periods of rest. In inflammatory arthritis, it can last for several hours and in some cases return at the end of the day. Don't forget that in well controlled rheumatoid arthritis, the lack of inflammation may result in stiffness lasting less than 30 minutes
- Swelling – intermittent swelling is suggestive of inflammatory arthritis. Swelling isolated to the knee is more likely to be non-inflammatory in nature. Ankle swelling may be oedema
- Pattern recognition – rheumatoid arthritis tends to be polyarticular, symmetrically affect the peripheral joints (sparing the distal interphalangeal joints). Psoriatic arthritis does affect the distal interphalangeal joints and is often asymmetrical. Osteoarthritis is more common in weight bearing joints or those prone to overuse (such as the first carpometacarpal joint)
- Other features – other system involvement is a clear pointer towards inflammatory arthropathies, whereas osteoarthritis is limited to the musculoskeletal system
- Psoriasis – you will look silly if you don't ask about or look for it! Bear in mind that the patient themselves may only have noticed dandruff
- Be aware of something known as palindromic rheumatism, which is an atypical presentation of recurrent short attacks of mono- or oligoarthritis which resolve spontaneously without any residual damage. Such patients are much more likely to go on to develop rheumatoid arthritis
- Finally – just because a patient has osteoarthritis, this does not mean they cannot develop a secondary problem such as a crystal arthropathy or even rheumatoid arthritis

RHEUMATOID ARTHRITIS

Rheumatoid arthritis (RA) is a chronic, systemic, inflammatory disease of unknown aeitiology that primarily affects the peripheral joints in a symmetrical pattern.

EPIDEMIOLOGY

- Prevalence is 1-3%
- There is a female to male ratio of 3:1
- Onset is at any age, but peaks in the 40's
- Occurs across all ethnic groups, but is rarer in Chinese and Japanese populations
- Associated with HLA DR4

PATIENT ASSESSMENT

- Classically there is a gradual onset of pain, stiffness and swelling symmetrically affecting the peripheral joints (sparing the DIP joints)
- Stiffness is worse in the morning and after rest
- Symptoms lasting for at least 6 weeks

Key musculoskeletal features
- Tender, boggy synovitis
- Ulnar deviation of the MCPs
- Swan neck and Boutonniere deformities
- 'Z' deformity of the thumb
- Trigger finger/tendon rupture
- Hallux valgus and hammer toes
- MTP involvement ('walking on pebbles')
- Ankle deformity is rare (it is a mortise joint)

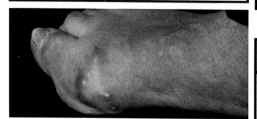

In some locations, nodules can be very problematic

INVESTIGATIONS

- Raised inflammatory markers, low albumin and raised ALP are common in active disease
- Anaemia (is multifactorial)
- Rheumatoid factor (RhF) is positive in 70%
- Anti-cyclic citrullinated peptide (anti-CCP) antibody has a specificity of 95%
- X-ray findings include a loss of joint space, soft tissue swelling, bony erosions, peri-articular osteopenia and subluxation

ACR/EULAR CRITERIA

- The traditional 1987 American College of Rheumatology criteria had been criticised for its lack of sensitivity in early disease
- Therefore in 2010, the American College of Rheumatology (ACR) and European League Against Rheumatism (EULAR) developed a new approach to classifying RA
- The classification is split into four categories (A-D), and a total score of six or more (out of ten) indicates 'definite rheumatoid arthritis'
A – Joint involvement (score of 0-5)
B – Serology (score of 0-3)
C – Acute phase reactants (score of 0-1)
D – Duration of symptoms (score of 0-1)

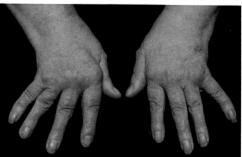

Classical rheumatoid hands

ADDITIONAL FEATURES

Extra-articular features
- Nodules (in 25% of cases, all RhF positive)
- Eye involvement. Keratoconjunctivitis sicca, episcleritis (red and painless) and scleritis (red and painful) are most common
- Secondary Sjögren's syndrome
- Cardiorespiratory features (common, but often asymptomatic)
- Increased risk of ischaemic heart disease
- Neurological, especially carpel tunnel syndrome
- Vasculitis
- Osteoporosis
- Depression
- Systemic effects such as malaise and fever
- Increased susceptibility to infections
- Rarely, Felty syndrome or amyloidosis

RHEUMATOID ARTHRITIS

MANAGEMENT BASICS

- Physiotherapy and occupational therapy, including aids for everyday activities
- Patient education and support groups
- Analgesia
- Disease modifying antirheumatic drugs DMARDs (e.g. methotrexate and sulfasalazine)
- Steroids (useful as a 'bridging' therapy when starting DMARDs and for flares). For severe flares, intravenous steroids may be used
- Biological therapies (e.g. anti-TNF therapy)
- Surgery in selected patients
- Management of cardiovascular risk factors

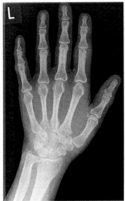 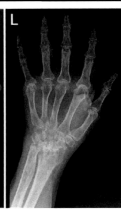

NICE GUIDELINES ON MANAGEMENT (2009)

- Treatment with DMARDs should begin as soon as possible after diagnosis to prevent further damage. NICE recommends combination therapy with methotrexate, at least one other DMARD and short term steroids (it takes 3 months to get maximal benefit from DMARDs)
- If combination therapy is not appropriate, the focus of monotherapy should be on achieving a clinically effective dose as soon as possible
- Once the disease is stable, DMARDs can be cautiously reduced, but should be re-increased at the first sign of a flare.
- Monthly measurements of disease activity (e.g. with DAS28) are recommended until control of disease is achieved
- Patients should have access to an MDT member who can co-ordinate care
- Steroids can be offered for short term use during flares, and should only be used as long term therapy when the risks and side effects have been discussed with the patient
- Paracetamol and codeine are first line analgesics for RA. NSAIDs and COX-2 inhibitors should be used at the minimal effective dose with a proton pump inhibitor only after their potential side effects have been considered

- Blood test monitoring whilst taking DMARDS is extremely important
- It is important to discuss activities such as diving due to involvement of the cervical spine

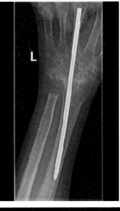

X-rays showing the progression from early very minimal changes to clear joint space reduction, periarticular osteopenia, soft tissue swelling and erosions. The same patient then underwent one of the more simple (but effective) surgical procedures for RA; excision of the lateral end of the ulna and arthrodesis of the wrist with an intramedullary nail

SELF ASSESSMENT

A 42 year old lady is referred by her GP with symmetrical pain, swelling and tenderness of her MCP and PIP joints. On examination she has active synovitis and nodules. You diagnose rheumatoid arthritis.

- You order blood tests, what is the probability that she is rheumatoid factor positive?
- You have obtained normal baseline blood test results, give an example of an appropriate drug regime?
- Six months later, she develops a red eye. There is no pain or itch and her vision is normal. What is the most likely cause?
- At the same review, you note that she is anaemic. Can you list any potential explanations?
- At a later review she complains that she is finding it difficult to swallow food. What else should you ask her and what is the most likely explanation?
- You also order hand x-rays, what changes will you be looking for?

SYSTEMIC LUPUS ERYTHEMATOSUS

Systemic lupus erythematosus (SLE) is a chronic, autoimmune, inflammatory, multisystem, connective tissue disorder that can affect almost any system in the body.

EPIDEMIOLOGY

- Classically affects women of child bearing age (20-40)
- There is a female:male ratio of 10:1
- More common in Afro-Caribbean, Asian and Hispanic communities
- There has been a significant rise in incidence over the last half century
- Associated with HLA B8, DR2 and DR3

PATIENT ASSESSMENT

- As SLE is a multi-system disorder, it is vitally important to enquire about and examine multiple systems, particularly the features listed below and potential triggers

ADDITIONAL FEATURES

It is important to remember that there is considerable variation in disease severity and organ involvement

- Systemic features (fever, fatigue, etc.)
- Arthralgia/arthritis (non-erosive)
- Myalgia
- Rash (photosensitive, malar, discoid or vasculitic)
- Oral and nasal ulcers
- Alopecia
- Raynaud's phenomenon
- Renal involvement, particularly signs and symptoms of glomerulonephritis (the kidneys are the most common organ to be affected)
- Neurological features (including headaches especially migraines, psychosis, seizures and depression)
- Haematological features include haemolytic anaemia, leucopenia, lymphopenia and thrombocytopenia. Anaemia may also be of chronic disease
- Cardiorespiratory serositis. Libman Sacks endocarditis, myocarditis, and shrinking lung syndrome may also occur
- Gastrointestinal features
- Eye involvement (keratoconjunctivitis sicca, anterior uveitis or may be secondary to hydroxychloroquine)
- Features of secondary Sjögren's or antiphospholipid syndrome (APS)

AEITIOLOGY

- There is evidence for genetic, environmental and hormonal influences in the aeitiology of SLE (that are beyond the scope of this book)
- There are several factors that are implicated in triggering flares, including overexposure to sunlight, oestrogen containing contraceptives, infections and stress
- There are a number of immunological abnormalities including immune complex formation and impaired clearance from tissues, a high ratio of CD4+ to CD8+ T cells, dysfunctional signalling and loss of immune tolerance leading to formation of autoantibodies
- There is a drug induced form of lupus

  It is more common in men than women

  Offending drugs include tetracyclines, hydralazine, procainamide, isoniazid, chlorpromazine, methyldopa and phenytoin

  100% are ANA positive and anti-double stranded DNA (dsDNA) antibody negative

  It is less severe than SLE, only rarely has renal and neurological involvement and should resolve on stopping the offending drug
- Additionally, discoid lupus, a benign disorder without the systemic features of SLE, tends to affect younger females, is classically characterised by follicular keratin plugs and in 5% progresses to SLE

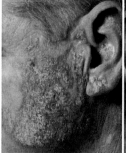
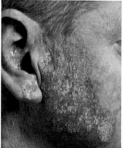
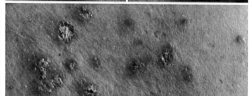

A gentleman with discoid lupus

SYSTEMIC LUPUS ERYTHEMATOSUS

INVESTIGATIONS

- Full blood count (see haematological features)
- ESR is indicative of disease activity. CRP is often normal except in arthritis, serositis or concurrent infection
- ANA has a sensitivity of 98% (but poor specificity). Anti-dsDNA antibodies are highly specific (99%), but less sensitive (70%) and are useful in disease monitoring in those that are positive.
- Anti-smith antibodies are the most specific (>99%), but even less sensitive (around 30%)
- 25% of patients are rheumatoid factor positive
- Compliment (C3, C4) levels are low when there is disease activity (consumed as complexes are formed). Low levels are also suggestive of renal disease
- Screening for renal disease, including blood pressure checks, U&Es and urinalysis for protein, red cells and casts
- If APTT is prolonged, it should prompt checking of antiphospholipid antibodies
- Anticardiolipin antibodies and lupus anticoagulant may be positive if there is associated antiphospholipid syndrome
- Direct Coombs test is often positive and classically there is a biologic false positive serological test for syphilis (not routine tests)
- CT/MRI head, cardiac echo or a renal biopsy can be useful if particular organ involvement is suspected

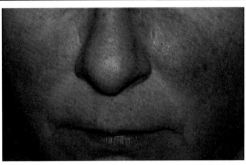

A malar rash, classically sparing the nasolabial folds (photo used with permission from cure4lupus.org)

- SLE sufferers are at increased risk of atherosclerosis, hypertension, dyslipidaemia, diabetes, osteoporosis, avascular necrosis, permanent neurological damage and lymphoma

MANAGEMENT BASICS

Depends upon severity and organs involved
- Patient education, including advice about avoiding sunlight and use of sunscreens, diet, smoking cessation, exercise and planning pregnancies carefully
- Cardiovascular risk reduction
- NSAIDs for symptomatic relief
- Steroids and antimalarials
- Other immunosuppressive agents such as cyclophosphamide, azathioprine and methotrexate are used when there is major organ involvement (note that sulfasalazine is avoided as it is linked to drug induced lupus)
- Rituximab is useful in severe disease (but is unlicensed for this indication)
- Plasma exchange is an option for aggressive and life threatening SLE

SELF ASSESSMENT

A GP refers a 35 year old lady to you in the rheumatology clinic with a photosensitive rash, Raynaud's phenomenon and some aches and pains in the joints of the hand. You suspect SLE.
- What other symptoms should you ask about?
- Which blood tests should you request?
- If her ANA comes back as negative, could she still have SLE?
- What haematological abnormalities might be seen in a patient with SLE?
- In fact her ANA, dsDNA antibodies and anti-sm antibodies are all positive and this confirms the diagnosis of SLE. What advice would you give her about triggers of disease activity?
- Which blood tests can be used to monitor disease activity in this patient?
- What is the most commonly affected organ in SLE and what therefore must you do at every follow up appointment?
- If you performed hand x-rays on this lady, what type of erosions might you see?

You then see a male patient who has developed some cutaneous symptoms whilst taking minocycline and is ANA positive. You suspect drug induced lupus.
- Which organs are classically spared?
- What is the key management step?

PSORIATIC ARTHRITIS

Psoriatic arthritis (PsA) is a chronic seronegative inflammatory arthritis associated with psoriasis. As with rheumatoid arthritis, PsA is characterised by flares and remissions.

EPIDEMIOLOGY

- 1.5% of the UK population has psoriasis
- PsA occurs in around 10% of these patients
- Additionally 15% of patients develop the arthritis before the psoriasis
- There is a peak of onset between the ages of 35 and 55, although it can occur at any age
- Even though psoriasis affects males and females equally, PsA is slightly more common in females (except for the spondylitic and distal interphalangeal forms)
- It is much more common in western, Caucasian populations
- It is associated with HLA-B27

PATIENT ASSESSMENT

- Overall, peripheral joint arthritis occurs in 95% of cases (exclusive axial spine involvement occurs in the other 5%)
- A diagnosis can be made without a history of psoriasis if there is a characteristic pattern and a family history of psoriasis
- Distal (and proximal) interphalangeal involvement is more common than metacarpophalangeal or metatarsophalangeal involvement
- A relapsing and remitting pattern is common, which does not necessarily correlate with the activity of the skin disease
- On examination it is important to check for psoriasis in 'hidden' areas such as the hairline, particularly behind the ears, the umbilicus and in the natal cleft

PATTERNS OF DISEASE

1. Symmetrical polyarthritis (or rheumatoid pattern)
- Mainly affects wrists, hands, feet and ankles
- Distal interphalangeal (DIP) joints are most frequently affected, helping to distinguish it from rheumatoid arthritis. Other differences are less deformity, lack of nodules and negative serology (RhF and anti-CCP)
2. Asymmetric oligoarthritis
- Mainly affects hands and feet
- Dactylitis (sausage fingers) is a key feature
- Usually less than five joints are affected
3. Lone DIP disease
- Primarily affects men
- Nail and paronychial involvement is common
4. Spondylitic pattern
- Can occur with or without sacroiliitis
- Presents with morning stiffness and restricted spinal movement
- Vertebrae are usually affected asymmetrically (distinguishing it from ankylosing spondylitis)
- The atlantoaxial joint may also be involved
5. Arthritis mutilans
- A rarer form, but most destructive
- Telescoping of fingers and the pencil in cup deformity (on x-rays) are important features
6. Juvenile onset
- Accounts for 10-20% of childhood arthritis
- Monoarthritis and DIP joint presentations are most common
- Tenosynovitis, nail changes and epiphyseal plate problems (stunting growth) are common

ADDITIONAL FEATURES

- Nail changes include pitting, yellowing, onycholysis, Beau lines, leukonychia and transverse ridging
- Extra-articular features are less common than in rheumatoid arthritis, but the most common are ocular involvement (uveitis or conjunctivitis) and entheses of the Achilles tendon
- The presence of subcutaneous nodules with psoriatic skin lesions and arthritis should raise the possibility of separate diagnoses of psoriasis and rheumatoid arthritis rather than psoriatic arthritis

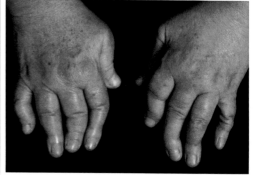

Hands of a patient with PsA. It can often be difficult to clinically distinguish from rheumatoid arthritis

PSORIATIC ARTHRITIS

INVESTIGATIONS

- Routine blood tests
- Inflammatory markers may be raised
- Rheumatoid factor is usually negative, but a positive result does not exclude PsA (just as a positive rheumatoid factor does not equal rheumatoid arthritis)
- IgA may be elevated
- Synovial fluid often contains large numbers of white blood cells
- Characteristic x-ray changes include bone erosions at the cartilage edge, a pencil in cup deformity and nonmarginal unilateral spinal syndesmophytes. Also of note is the absence of periarticular osteopenia and less symmetry than in rheumatoid arthritis

A hand x-ray suggestive of inflammatory arthritis; the DIP joint involvement and absence of peri-articular osteopenia should raise the possibility of psoriatic arthritis

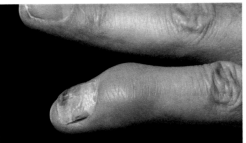

DIP joint involvement and nail changes are classical of psoriatic arthritis

- Despite having a better prognosis than rheumatoid arthritis, PsA can be just as destructive and also conveys an increased cardiovascular risk and therefore should be treated just as aggressively

MANAGEMENT BASICS

- Similar to that of rheumatoid arthritis
- Patient education
- Physiotherapy and occupational therapy
- Although NSAIDs can help the joints, they can worsen the skin psoriasis (as can hydroxychloroquine)
- Intra-articular steroids (there is a risk of rebound exacerbation of psoriasis with oral steroids)
- DMARDs, especially methotrexate and sulfasalazine
- Anti-TNF agents
- Retinoic-acid derivatives and psoralen plus ultraviolet light can have a beneficial effect on the arthritis as well as the skin
- Address risk factors for cardiovascular disease and metabolic syndrome

SELF ASSESSMENT

A 41 year old gentleman with a past medical history of psoriasis and "pains at the back of my ankle" is referred to the rheumatology clinic with pain and swelling of the joints of both hands.
- What percentage of patients with psoriasis go on to develop associated arthropathy?
- What are the key features from the history, examination and investigations that would point you towards a diagnosis of psoriatic rather than coincidental rheumatoid arthritis?
- In the context of psoriatic arthritis, can you explain the ankle pain?
- Whilst the management of psoriatic arthritis is similar to that of rheumatoid arthritis, some medications can lead to a flare of the skin disease. Can you name some?
- What is the 'pencil in cup' deformity and which other characteristic x-ray changes can you list?
- In a patient without known psoriasis, in which 'hidden' areas should you check?

GOUT

Gout is a disorder of uric acid metabolism resulting in bouts of arthropathy secondary to the deposition of crystals into the joints.

EPIDEMIOLOGY

- Has a prevalence of around 1% in the Caucasian population
- Much more common in men and advancing age
- Rare in premenopausal women
- May be primary or secondary (see below)

CAUSES

PRIMARY
- Idiopathic (90% due to under-excretion of uric acid)
- Risk factors include increasing age, male sex, family history and obesity
- Gout in childhood may be secondary to an inherited metabolic disorder (such as Lesch–Nyhan syndrome)

SECONDARY
- Lifestyle factors including foods rich in purines (oily fish, red meat), alcohol and extreme exercise.
- Hyperuricaemia
- Drugs (including diuretics, low dose aspirin, ciclosporin, alcohol, cytotoxic agents and pyrazinamide)
- Chronic renal failure
- Myeloproliferative/lymphoproliferative disorders
- Severe psoriasis
- Previous joint trauma
- Lead nephropathy
- Other predisposing conditions include hypertension, diabetes mellitus, ischaemic heart disease and hypothyroidism

ADDITIONAL FEATURES

- Tophi are when the yellow/ivory urate crystals can be seen through the skin
- These tophi can ulcerate or a secondary infection may occur
- Urate nephropathy including urate stone formation. End stage renal failure can occur if chronic gout is left untreated
- Avascular necrosis of the femoral head
- Rarely, nerve entrapment (e.g. carpal tunnel syndrome) or spinal cord compression

PATIENT ASSESSMENT

- The symptoms of an acutely red, hot, tender, swollen painful joint, with a reduced range of movement peak at around 24 hours and last for up to two weeks
- Ask about lifestyle, predisposing conditions, medications and previous episodes
- 70% of first and 50% of all presentations affect the 1st metatarsophalangeal joint
- Fever and malaise may occur
- The patient is usually asymptomatic between attacks
- Tophi, (look particularly at the hands, feet, elbows and ears), classically occur in chronic gout in post menopausal women on diuretic therapy
- Chronic gout can be poly- or oligoarticular and is often asymmetrical

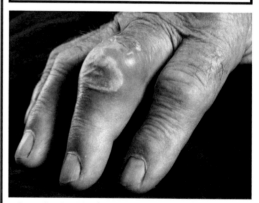

Gout affecting the 3rd PIP joint with a large tophi

INVESTIGATIONS

- The gold standard is the demonstration of negatively birefringent needle shaped crystals in synovial fluid
- Fluid should also be sent for gram stain and culture (as sepsis may co-exist)
- Urate level (very limited diagnostic value)
- Inflammatory markers and routine blood tests
- Glucose and lipid profile (risk factors)
- X-rays are usually unhelpful in acute gout, but can show punched out erosions and/or subcortical cysts in chronic disease

GOUT

MANAGEMENT BASICS

Acute attack
- NSAIDs
- If the symptoms fail to settle, colchicine or steroids (often intra-articular) are next line
- Analgesia

Prophylaxis of chronic gout
- Lifestyle modification. For example weight loss if obese, reduce alcohol and purine intake, regular exercise, smoking cessation and avoiding dehydration
- Indications for medical prophylaxis include recurrent attacks (two or more within 12 months), tophi, renal disease, chemotherapy, diuretic treatment or Lesch-Nyhan syndrome
- Medication review
- Treat associated diabetes, hyperlipidaemia or hypertension
- Allopurinol (a xanthine oxidase inhibitor), is first line, but is only routinely started 2-4 weeks after an acute episode
- Other drugs that are sometimes used in chronic gout include febuxostat, probenecid, sulfinpyrazone & benzbromarone. Long term colchicine may be considered but there is a risk of neuromyopathy
- Losartan, amlodipine, atorvastatin and fenofibrate also have uricosuric effects
- Surgery may be considered for large or ulcerated tophi

- Uricosuric drugs should be avoided in patients with renal impairment and/or stones

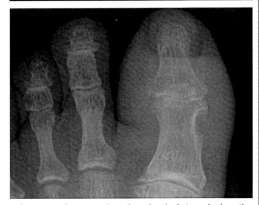

An x-ray demonstrating the classical 'punched out' erosion away from the joint margin

PSEUDOGOUT

- Pseudogout is caused by the deposition of calcium pyrophosphate crystals in joints
- The patterns include asymptomatic, acute monoarthritis, inflammatory arthritis or secondary osteoarthritis
- Knee, wrist, shoulders and hips are most commonly affected
- The main risk factors are dehydration, haemochromatosis, hyperparathyroidism, low magnesium or phosphate, hypothyroidism and Wilson's disease
- Joint aspiration classically shows weakly positively birefringent rhomboid shaped crystals
- X-rays often show chondrocalcinosis
- Management is only in symptomatic cases and includes excluding septic arthritis, NSAIDs, steroids and correction of any metabolic disturbance

SELF ASSESSMENT

A 61 year old man with a background of stage 3 renal failure secondary to type 1 diabetes mellitus presents with a painful, red swollen left knee. Even though you would want to exclude septic arthritis, you suspect a crystal arthropathy.
- What is the main causative factor of gout?
- You examine his hands but can't see any tophi. Where else should you specifically look? Why might you not see any in this patient?
- If this was pseudogout, what might you see on his x-ray?
- You aspirate his joint, and on microscopy you see needle shaped crystals and no organisms. Given the diagnosis, what would be the most appropriate initial therapy? What is the main side effect?
- Why might his urate level be normal?
- Which joint would have been more classical for a first presentation?
- On discharge what general advice should you give him?
- How many further attacks in the next 12 months does he need to have before you start prophylaxis, and which agent would you use?
- This gentleman goes on to have chronic gout, particularly affecting his hands and feet. What are the key x-ray findings you might see (or not see)?

You are asked to review a different gentleman with a raised urate level, who is asymptomatic.
- Should you offer him treatment?

OSTEOPOROSIS

Osteoporosis is the progressive loss of bone density resulting in bone fragility and therefore an increased risk of fracture.

EPIDEMIOLOGY

- Most commonly affects post menopausal women (50% of women aged over 70)
- NICE estimates that there are 2 million women with osteoporosis in the UK
- It causes over 300,000 fractures a year in the UK
- More common in Caucasians (and Asians) than in Afro-Caribbean individuals

PATIENT ASSESSMENT

- Often asymptomatic until fractures occur
- The key is to recognise 'low trauma fragility fractures'

Common sites of fracture
- The femoral neck (severe pain and shortening and external rotation of the leg)
- Vertebrae (spinal tenderness on percussion and kyphosis and loss of height if multiple fractures have occurred)
- Distal radius (dinner fork deformity of a Colles' fracture after falling onto an outstretched hand)
- Humerus

CAUSES

Primary
- Post menopausal
- Idiopathic
- Osteoporosis of pregnancy

Secondary
- Endocrine causes including hypogonadism (testosterone deficiency is an important cause in middle aged men), Cushing syndrome, hypopituitarism, hyperthyroidism and primary hyperparathyroidism
- Medications such as steroids and long term heparin therapy
- Malignancy, particularly multiple myeloma, metastatic carcinoma and leukaemia
- Rheumatological causes such as rheumatoid arthritis and ankylosing spondylitis
- Gastrointestinal conditions including coeliac disease, inflammatory bowel disease, primary biliary sclerosis and post gastrectomy
- Other causes include chronic renal failure, osteogenesis imperfecta and homocystinuria

RISK FACTORS

- Increasing age
- Family history
- Female sex
- Low body mass index
- Anorexia nervosa
- Poor diet (especially low calcium and vitamin D intake)
- Low exposure to sunlight
- Sedentary lifestyle
- Smoking
- Alcohol intake of four or more units a day
- Untreated premature menopause
- Late menarche
- Prolonged secondary amenorrhoea
- Mulitparity

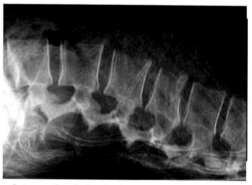

Osteoporotic spinal wedge fracture

INVESTIGATIONS

- Bone densitometry with a dual-energy x-ray absorptiometry (DEXA) scan is the gold standard for diagnosis
- Calcium, phosphate and alkaline phosphatase levels are normal (if abnormal there is likely to be a secondary cause or a recent fracture)
- Routine and specific blood tests to investigate for secondary causes
- A testosterone level should always be checked in men
- X-rays to diagnose fractures. Over 30% loss of bone density is needed before radiolucency is evident

OSTEOPOROSIS

MANAGEMENT BASICS

- Patient education
- Weight bearing exercises
- Hip protectors
- Reduce polypharmacy and other risk factors for falls
- Treat any secondary cause
- Ensure adequate calcium and vitamin D intake (supplement if necessary)
- Advice regarding smoking cessation and reducing alcohol intake
- Hormone replacement therapy in post menopausal women (but it is not recommended for long term use due to risks of cardiovascular disease and breast cancer)
- Bisphosphonates are the mainstay for both treatment and prevention of osteoporosis
- Examples of bisphosphonates include alendronate, risedronate, etidronate and zoledronate
- Testosterone if appropriate in men
- Selective oestrogen receptor modulators (SERMs, e.g. raloxifene) can also reduce the risk of breast cancer, but should not be used first line
- Other drug treatments for osteoporosis include strontium ranelate, parathyroid hormone peptides, denosumab and calcitonin (although the latter's effect is limited to the vertebrae)

- The epidemiological data equates to an osteoporotic fracture every 2-3 minutes in the UK
- The mortality of a hip fracture in the elderly is 20% at 3 months, and only 50% of survivors regain full independence

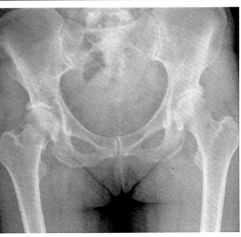

There is obvious evidence of osteoporosis on this pelvis x-ray. There is also a right sided femoral neck fracture

DEXA SCAN RESULTS

- When bone density is measured it is expressed as a T score and a Z score
- A T score is the number of standard deviations the patient's bone density is away from the optimal density for their sex
- A Z score is the number of standard deviations the patient's bone density is away from the age, sex, weight and ethnicity matched normal
- The T score is used to define osteoporosis
- The Z score can be useful in identifying those that may have a secondary cause of their osteoporosis
- A normal T score is above -1
- A T score between −1 and −2.5 represents osteopenia
- A T score below −2.5 is diagnostic of osteoporosis
- Severe osteoporosis is defined as a T score below −2.5 and a fragility fracture

SELF ASSESSMENT

A 48 year old man has back pain. X-rays reveal vertebral collapse and osteoporosis. He has no significant medical history.
- What lifestyle factors should you ask him about?
- What key blood test should you request for a middle-aged man?

A 70 year old man has previously been diagnosed with polymyalgia rheumatica. You note that he is taking 10mg of prednisolone.
- You are rightly concerned about osteoporosis. Would calcium with vitamin D supplements or a bisphosphonate be most appropriate?
- Should you perform a DEXA scan?
- Other than steroids, can you name another drug that can cause osteoporosis?

A 50 year old lady with a background of rheumatoid arthritis, who has had numerous courses of prednisolone has a DEXA scan. Her femoral neck T score = -1.9.
- What does this T score mean?
- What treatment would be most appropriate?

SYSTEMIC SCLEROSIS

Systemic sclerosis (SSc) is a multisystem, connective tissue disease, characterised by increased fibrosis of tissues.

EPIDEMIOLOGY

- Incidence is 4-12 per million per year
- Seen in all ethnic groups across the globe
- There is a female:male ratio of 4:1
- Can present at any age, but the peak is between 25-55 years and is rare in children

PATIENT ASSESSMENT

- Hands for swelling (non pitting oedema), sclerodactyly (hard and thickened skin), flexion deformities, tendon friction rubs, calcinosis and finger tip ulcers secondary to Raynaud's phenomenon
- Generally for telangiectasia, the salt-and-pepper appearance of hyperpigmentation and hypopigmentation (particularly over the lower legs) and tightening of skin
- Enquire about smoking and nutrition

ADDITIONAL FEATURES

- Raynaud's phenomenon
- Musculoskeletal: Arthralgia (erosive arthritis occurs in 30% of patients) and myositis
- Respiratory: Pulmonary fibrosis leading to pulmonary hypertension
- Renal: Hypertensive renal crisis progressing to renal failure
- Gastrointestinal: Dry mouth, oesophageal dysmotility (motility can be impaired at any level), reflux oesophagitis, watermelon stomach, malabsorption (due to bacterial overgrowth), pseudo-obstruction and constipation (due to chronic hypomotility)
- Cardiac: Pericarditis, pericardial effusion, myocardial fibrosis, cardiac failure and arrhythmias
- Others: Trigeminal neuralgia, impotence and hypothyroidism

RENAL CRISIS

- Usually presents with features of accelerated hypertension and is a serious complication
- More common with diffuse disease
- Treatment is with ACE inhibitors. Dialysis may be required in some cases

SUBSETS OF SSc

Limited cutaneous systemic sclerosis
- Generally milder than the diffuse form (70% 10 year survival), with a slower onset
- Skin involvement is often limited to the face, neck and distal parts of limbs
- Raynaud's phenomenon is often the first sign
- Pulmonary hypertension is more common than renal crisis
- CREST (calcinosis, Raynaud's phenomenon, oesophageal dysmotility, sclerodactyly and telangiectasia) is a subtype of the limited form of the disease

Diffuse cutaneous systemic sclerosis
- More severe than the limited form (50% 10 year survival), with a significantly faster onset of symptoms, but does tend to become more stable after a few years
- Skin involvement is more widespread
- Internal organ involvement is more common
- Finger swelling is often the first sign
- Renal crisis is more common than pulmonary hypertension

Scleroderma (with no internal involvement)
- Morphoea (plaques)
- En coup de sabre (linear lesions of the scalp and face, with underlying bone changes)

Scleroderma sine scleroderma
- Internal organ involvement, with no skin changes

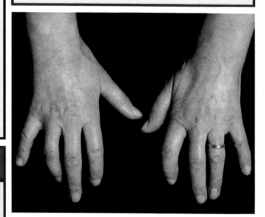

This lady has systemic sclerosis. Note the shininess of the skin and the finger swelling, particularly of the 2nd digit of her left hand

SYSTEMIC SCLEROSIS

INVESTIGATIONS

- Routine bloods tests may show elevated inflammatory markers, renal impairment, anaemia and thrombocytopenia
- 30% of patients are rheumatoid factor positive
- 90% of patients are antinuclear antibody positive
- Anti-Scl70 and RNA-polymerase are associated with diffuse systemic sclerosis, whilst anti-centromere antibodies are associated with the limited form of the condition
- There are other auto-antibodies involved that are discussed further on page 30
- Urine protein:creatinine ratio
- Nailfold capillaroscopy
- Hand x-ray (may show calcinosis)
- Specific investigations for other associated features

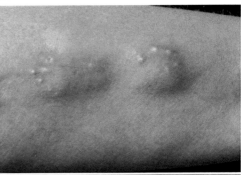
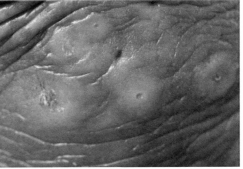

Calcinosis does not only occur in the fingers. This patient had calcinosis of the forearm (top) and just below her knees (bottom) as well as on the tip of her nose (not shown)

MANAGEMENT BASICS

- Patient education and explanation
- Physiotherapy, home exercises and occupational therapy
- Smoking, weight and nutritional advice
- Camouflage products and moisturisers for the skin
- Penicillamine can slow the progression of skin disease (but steroids do not help, and may increase the risk of renal crisis)
- Steroids and other immunosuppressive agents for pulmonary fibrosis
- ACE inhibitors can reduce the incidence of renal crisis, which if occurs may require dialysis
- Proton pump inhibitors for reflux symptoms
- Prokinetic drugs such as domperidone may improve oesophageal motility
- Surgery can be used to release contractures or remove any problematic calcinosis
- Plus treatments for specific complications

- Systemic sclerosis is more severe in non-Caucasian patients. Male sex is also a poor prognostic factor
- There are overlap syndromes with SLE and polymyositis

SELF ASSESSMENT

You review in clinic a 47 year old lady with the diagnosis of CREST.
- What does CREST stand for?
- Which of the five features is she most likely to have developed first?

You also review a lady of the same age with diffuse cutaneous systemic sclerosis.
- Is she likely to have a better or worse prognosis than the lady with CREST?
- She complains of symptoms of malabsorption. Why does this occur in systemic sclerosis?
- Is she more likely to develop pulmonary hypertension or renal crisis?
- What non-drug management advice could you offer her?
- Why should high dose steroids be avoided in a patient with diffuse cutaneous systemic sclerosis?
- How can surgery have a role in patients with systemic sclerosis?
- Watermelon stomach is listed in the additional features section, but what is it?

RAYNAUD'S PHENOMENON

Raynaud's phenomenon (RP) is a relatively common disorder characterised by triphasic colour changes of fingers, toes and sometimes other parts of the body.

EPIDEMIOLOGY

- RP is very common with up to 15% of the adult population of the UK being affected, but most do not consult a doctor
- It is much more common in women
- Risk factors include smoking, vibrating tools and particularly in women, family history and oestrogen exposure
- Cold weather and emotional stress are common triggers

PATIENT ASSESSMENT

- Details of the symptoms
- Triggers and relieving factors
- The use of a diary and photography during an attack can be useful
- Symptoms of potential secondary causes (including migraines, joint pains, rashes, ulcers, dysphagia and xerostomia)
- Occupation, medications, smoking status and family history are also important
- Examination should focus upon assessing the hands and feet for signs of tissue damage and for signs of potential secondary causes

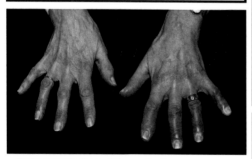

The hyperaemic phase of Raynaud's phenomenon

ADDITIONAL FEATURES

- The main secondary causes of RP are connective tissue diseases, peripheral vascular disease and thoracic outlet syndrome.
- Associated features and complications would therefore be specific to the individual cause

INVESTIGATIONS

- Routine blood tests including inflammatory markers and thyroid function tests
- A full immunology screen is often requested, although it is the anti-nuclear antibody (ANA) that is the key component due to its association with connective tissue diseases
- Further tests depend upon potential causes and include a chest x-ray for a cervical rib
- Nailfold capillaroscopy is becoming increasingly utilised and can be performed with an ophthalmoscope

MANAGEMENT BASICS

- Patient education, including advice about triggers such as cold weather. This extends to the use of heated clothing to maintain core temperature
- Smoking cessation
- Hand and feet exercises can reduce the frequency of attacks by improving circulation
- Vasodilators, such as calcium channel blockers (nifedipine is first line), topical nitrates, prostaglandins (particularly iloprost), phosphodiesterase type 5 inhibitors (Sildenafil) and antioxidants
- Inhibitors of vasoconstriction, for example, angiotensin receptor antagonists (losartan) and Endothelin receptor antagonists (bosentan)
- Beta-blockers should be avoided
- Surgery is occasionally considered in refractory cases

OTHER KEY POINTS

- Attacks usually last from minutes to hours. In addition to the hands and feet, the ears, nose, tongue and jaw can be affected

SELF ASSESSMENT

- What is the difference between primary and secondary RP?
- What general advice can you give to a patient with RP?
- Which antihypertensive should be avoided?

SJOGREN'S SYNDROME

Sjögren's Syndrome is a chronic autoimmune disorder, characterised by lymphocytic infiltration of exocrine glands resulting in dry mucous membranes.

EPIDEMIOLOGY

- Sjögren's syndrome is very common with a prevalence of up to 4% of the UK population
- There is a female:male ratio of 9:1
- Onset is usually between the ages of 30-60
- May be primary or secondary to connective tissue disorders (e.g. rheumatoid arthritis or SLE) or organ specific autoimmune diseases (e.g. primary biliary cirrhosis, autoimmune hepatitis or autoimmune thyroid disease)
- In Caucasians there is an association with HLA-B8 and HLA-DR3

INVESTIGATIONS

- Routine blood tests (anaemia is common)
- Elevated amylase and inflammatory markers
- ANA and rheumatoid factor are often positive
- In primary Sjögren's syndrome anti-Ro and anti-La antibodies are frequently positive
- Hypergammaglobulinaemia and low C4 levels may also be seen
- The Schirmer test can be used to detect dry eyes
- Biopsy of a salivary gland or lower lip may occasionally be performed

PATIENT ASSESSMENT

- The key feature is dryness of mucous membranes, especially the mouth, eyes, vagina and respiratory tract
- Ask patients about difficulty eating, change in taste, dental health, hoarseness, respiratory infections, dry skin, fatigue and dyspareunia
- On examination look under the tongue when checking for oral dryness
- History and examination should also focus upon the signs and symptoms of a secondary cause (in particular, connective tissue disorders)

MANAGEMENT BASICS

- Patient education, including promotion of good oral hygiene
- Artificial tears, lubricating gels at night and shielded spectacles for eye symptoms
- Artificial saliva sprays and mouthwashes
- Pilocarpine may stimulate saliva and tear production
- Hydroxychloroquine may be helpful for skin and joint symptoms
- Analgesia as required
- Emollients if dry skin is a problem

ADDITIONAL FEATURES

- A dry mouth can lead to dental caries and candidal infections
- Dry eyes can result in keratoconjunctivitis and corneal ulcers
- Other associated features include arthralgia (or erosive arthritis), dry skin, parotid gland swelling, lymphadenopathy, Raynaud's phenomenon, vasculitis, pancreatitis, sensory polyneuropathy, and renal tubular acidosis

- There is an increased incidence of mouth and eye infections
- At follow up appointments, patients should be examined for lymphadenopathy due to the risk of lymphoid malignancy

MALIGNANCY RISK

- Patients with Sjögren's syndrome have a marked increase in lymphoid malignancy (40-60 fold)
- Due to lymphocytic infiltration, up to 10% develop a lymphoproliferative disorder and 1% develop non-Hodgkin's lymphoma (the latter is associated with lower C4 counts)

SELF ASSESSMENT

You see a 39 year old lady with primary Sjögren's syndrome.
- Which two antibodies from the ENA screen are most likely to be positive?
- She has a Schirmer test. What is this?
- She continues to struggle with her dry mouth despite artificial saliva. Which medication could you try?

ANKYLOSING SPONDYLITIS

Ankylosing spondylitis (AS) is a chronic, multisystem inflammatory disorder that primarily affects sacroiliac joints and the axial skeleton.

EPIDEMIOLOGY

- AS has a prevalence of 0.15%
- The male:female ratio is 5:1
- The peak age onset is between 15 and 40
- Associated with HLA B27

PATIENT ASSESSMENT

The key features are
- Inflammatory back pain and stiffness
- Symptoms are worse in the early hours of the morning
- Improvement of symptoms with activity
- Sacroiliac joint tenderness
- Limited lateral flexion
- Then forward flexion (Schober's test)
- Reduced chest expansion
- A question mark posture in later stages

INFLAMMATORY PAIN

- Age of onset younger than 40
- Onset is insidious
- No improvement with rest
- Improvement with exercise
- Night pain (which improves on getting up)

BACK PAIN RED FLAGS

Features
- Previous malignancy (however long ago)
- Age under 16 or over 50 with new onset pain
- Unexplained weight loss
- Previous longstanding steroid use
- Other immunosuppression
- Recent serious illness or infection

Symptoms
- Non-mechanical pain
- Thoracic pain
- Fevers, rigors or general malaise
- Urinary retention

Signs
- Saddle anaesthesia or reduced anal tone
- Neurological deficit
- Progressive spinal deformity

ADDITIONAL FEATURES

Think about the 'A's
- Arthritis of peripheral joints (in 35%), more commonly in females
- Anterior uveitis (in 30%)
- Aortic regurgitation (in 4%)
- AV node block
- Achilles tendonitis
- Apical pulmonary fibrosis
- Amyloidosis
- And cauda equina syndrome

INVESTIGATIONS

- Anaemia and raised inflammatory markers and ALP are less common compared with other inflammatory conditions
- Rheumatoid factor is usually negative
- HLA-B27 has a limited diagnostic value as it is positive in 10% of the general population
- X-rays may show sclerosis, loss of lumbar lordosis, subchondral erosions, squaring of vertebrae with Romanus lesions, bamboo spine (syndesmophytes) and enthesitis
- MRI is having an increasing role

MANAGEMENT BASICS

- Patient education such as advice about sleeping flat on a firm mattress
- Physiotherapy and home exercises (including for breathing)
- NSAIDs
- DMARDs are only helpful for peripheral arthritis (sulfasalazine is commonly used)
- Anti-TNF therapy is effective
- Surgery for end stage disease

- Spirometry can show a restrictive pattern

SELF ASSESSMENT

- What is Schober's test?
- Which DMARD is most frequently used in AS?

OSTEOARTHRITIS

Osteoarthritis (OA) is by far the most common joint disorder. It is characterised by the destruction of cartilage, new bone formation and capsular fibrosis.

EPIDEMIOLOGY

- A quarter of those aged over 65 have symptomatic hip or knee OA
- 70% of 70 year olds have radiological evidence of OA
- Advancing age, family history, female sex (at least for knee OA), Caucasian ethnicity, joint injury, obesity and strenuous occupation are risk factors

PATIENT ASSESSMENT

- Joint pain is usually use related, occurring after activity. Stiffness, reduced range of movement, deformity and instability are also common
- Check for Heberden and Bouchard nodes (bony swellings at the DIP and PIP joints respectively)
- Joint effusions and crepitus on movement may be felt
- The most commonly affected joints are hips, knees, spine, first carpometacarpal joint, DIP joints and PIP joints

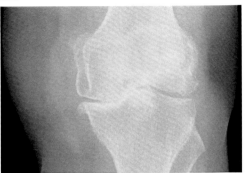
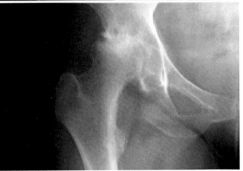

X-rays showing typical OA changes

ADDITIONAL FEATURES

- Systemic features are usually absent

INVESTIGATIONS

- Routine blood tests and immunology screen should be normal
- Joint aspirate is typically clear and viscous with low cell counts
- X-ray findings include joint space narrowing, subchondral cysts, subchondral sclerosis and osteophytes

SUBSETS OF OA

- Localised to one site
- Generalised
- Secondary to other disorders such as previous inflammation (RA, gout or sepsis), joint injury, inherited dysplastic disorders and some metabolic disorders

MANAGEMENT BASICS

- Patient education and advice about weight loss, local muscle strengthening exercises and aerobic fitness
- Physiotherapy and occupational therapy
- Supports and braces, thermotherapy and shock absorbing shoes can also be tried
- According to NICE, paracetamol and for knee or hand OA, topical NSAIDs are first line
- NSAIDs or COX-2 inhibitors (with a proton pump inhibitor) are second line
- Opioids can also be considered
- Intra-articular steroid injections are useful
- Surgical options include arthroscopy with debridement or replacement

SELF ASSESSMENT

- What do you know of the role of glucosamine?
- In which order would you try analgesics for a lady with knee OA?

PAGET'S DISEASE

Paget's disease is a disorder of bone remodelling. Increased activity from both osteoblasts and osteoclasts results in disorganised bone structure.

EPIDEMIOLOGY

- Paget's disease is rare in those aged under 40, but affects 5% of the elderly population
- The UK has the highest prevalence in the world and it is very rare in Asia
- There is a male:female ratio of 2:1
- 15% have a positive family history

PATIENT ASSESSMENT

- Most patients (95%) are asymptomatic. Diagnosis is made from incidental x-ray and biochemical findings
- Patients may present with bone pain; classically a constant dull ache, made worse by movement and weight bearing
- The most commonly affected sites are the pelvis, lumbar spine, femur and skull
- On examination look for the head signs (see images), warm skin overlying an affected part (increased vascularity), bowing of long bones (sabre tibia), and signs of the additional features below

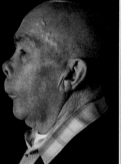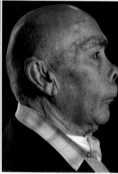

The skull features of Paget's disease include increased skull size, frontal bossing, deep set eyes due to a prominent orbital ridge and a large maxilla with prominent arches giving an increased distance between the nose and upper lip. The nostrils can also be misshaped.

ADDITIONAL FEATURES

- Other skeletal deformities such as a spinal kyphosis
- Pathological fractures (and pseudofractures)
- Secondary osteoarthritis
- Sensorineural deafness (due to compression of the vestibulocochlear nerve)
- Other neurological compression syndromes
- Osteosarcoma, spinal cord compression or high output cardiac failure can rarely occur

MANAGEMENT BASICS

- Walking sticks and orthotic devices
- Rest, then physiotherapy following stress fractures
- Paracetamol and NSAIDs for bone pain
- Medical treatment is indicated in those that are symptomatic, have complications or are close to developing complications
- The mainstay of treatment is with bisphosphonates (most commonly with oral risedronate or intravenous zoledronate)
- Calcitonin is now less frequently used
- Alkaline phosphate can be used to monitor the efficacy of treatment
- Surgery in certain cases, such as for nerve decompression, fracture fixation or joint replacements

INVESTIGATIONS

- Classically, there is a raised alkaline phosphatase, with normal phosphate and calcium levels (the latter, however, can rise following immobilisation)
- In patients with abnormal liver function, bone specific alkaline phosphate can be requested
- The key x-ray finding is enlarged, deformed bones with mixed sclerotic and lytic areas
- A 'cotton wool' skull pattern, and blade of grass 'V' shaped lesion of long bones are classical

- Patients require long term follow up even if they respond well to treatment due to the risk of osteosarcoma

SELF ASSESSMENT

- What percentage of patients with Paget's disease are symptomatic at presentation?
- Which bones are most frequently affected?
- What is the mainstay drug treatment?

POLYMYOSITIS & DERMATOMYOSITIS

Polymyositis is a symmetrical inflammatory disorder of skeletal muscle. It tends to affect proximal muscles. When associated with cutaneous features it is termed dermatomyositis.

EPIDEMIOLOGY

- It is rare; incidence is 5 cases per 100,000
- It is slightly more common in Afro-Caribbean individuals and in females. There is a small peak of presentation at 5-15 years of age and a larger peak at 40-65 years of age
- It may be idiopathic or associated with connective tissue diseases, vasculitis in childhood or underlying malignancy

PATIENT ASSESSMENT

- Patients present with progressive proximal weakness over 3-6 months
- Distal muscles are preserved until late
- About one-third have myalgia or arthralgia

Additional features of dermatomyositis
- Purple heliotrope rash on upper eyelids with periorbital oedema
- Macular rash, particularly over the upper back, shoulders and chest (shawl sign)
- Erythema of the extensor surface of joints, especially the elbows and knees
- Gottron's papules over finger joints
- Nailfold capillary dilatation

ADDITIONAL FEATURES

- Fatigue, malaise, fever and weight loss
- Dysphagia due to pharyngeal weakness
- Pulmonary muscle weakness
- Interstitial pulmonary disease
- Raynaud's phenomenon

INVESTIGATIONS

- Creatine kinase can be massively raised
- AST and LDH are also elevated
- ANA is positive in 60%
- Anti-Jo1 antibodies are positive in a quarter of patients with polymyositis and are associated with a more acute onset, lung involvement, arthritis, fever and Raynaud's phenomenon and therefore a worse prognosis
- Electromyography (EMG) and muscle biopsy
- Due to the association with malignancy, tumour markers, imaging and faecal occult bloods should be considered

MANAGEMENT BASICS

- Patient education, physiotherapy and occupational therapy equipment
- Steroids are the mainstay of treatment. Response can be measured by creatine kinase levels, which tend to fall quickly, but muscle power often takes longer to improve
- Other immunosuppressive agents, which include azathioprine, cyclophosphamide or methotrexate may be used in resistant cases

- The average duration of active disease is 2-3 years and many have future exacerbations

SELF ASSESSMENT

You review a gentleman with dermatomyositis
- What characteristic skin lesions might you see?
- What is the likelihood that he is anti-Jo1 antibody positive?
- What serious association would you want to screen him for?

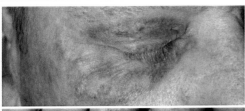
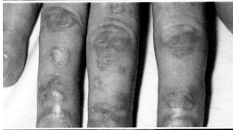
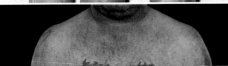

The heliotrope rash, Gottron's papules and shawl sign

SEPTIC ARTHRITIS

Septic arthritis is the inflammation of a joint secondary to infection. Both native or prosthetic joints can be affected.

EPIDEMIOLOGY

- Incidence is estimated to be 6 per 100,000 population per year
- The incidence in those with prosthetic joints is between 2-10%
- It is common in children as well as in adults
- It is becoming increasingly common in the elderly with multiple co-morbidities
- The most common organism overall is Staphylococcus aureus, although Neisseria gonorrhoeae should always be considered in young sexually active individuals
- Joint damage, such as from crystal arthropathies or rheumatoid arthritis, is an important risk factor

PATIENT ASSESSMENT

- Septic arthritis usually presents as hot, red, tender and swollen joint or joints (a single joint is affected in 85% of cases)
- Important points in the history include speed of onset, trauma, loss of function, number of joints that are affected and constitutional symptoms (fever, malaise, rigors etc.)
- Classically the patient will resist even small amounts of movement and are unable to weight bear
- Signs may be less obvious in the elderly and in those with prosthetic joints. It is therefore important to have a high index of suspicion in these patients

PATTERN OF INFECTION

- In adults, the most commonly affected joint is the knee (50% of cases). The wrists, hip, shoulder and ankles are also commonly affected
- In children, those younger than 3 years of age are affected most frequently. A third of cases affect the hip, a third the knee and a third the remaining joints
- The elbow, shoulder and ankle are the most frequently affected prosthetic joints
- In addition to the organisms mentioned above, streptococcal species are also common and the elderly are particularly vulnerable to gram-negative bacilli such as salmonella and pseudomonas

INVESTIGATIONS

- In any acutely hot, red and swollen joint, aspiration is the key investigation to exclude or confirm septic arthritis
- Joint aspirate should be sent for cell counts, gram stain, culture and microscopy (to check for crystals)
- Routine blood tests including inflammatory markers
- Immunology may be considered depending upon the presentation
- Blood cultures should also be taken to exclude bacteraemia
- X-rays are usually normal (but may show evidence of a differential diagnosis, e.g. gout). In more chronic cases x-rays can show evidence of osteomyelitis

MANAGEMENT BASICS

- Antibiotics for at least 6 weeks (initially intravenously). They should be started empirically whilst awaiting joint fluid analysis
- Repeated aspiration to decompress the joint may be required
- Orthopaedic review for consideration of 'wash out' ('the solution to pollution is dilution', or so they say)
- Regular review and examination of the joint affected and monitoring of inflammatory markers

- Mortality risk depends upon the causative organism. Staphylococcus aureus has significant mortality if treatment is delayed

SELF ASSESSMENT

You are asked to review a hot, red, swollen and tender joint. You suspect septic arthritis
- You aspirate the joint. What are the most important tests to request?
- What empirical treatment does the BNF advise whilst awaiting the results?
- Which joint is most commonly affected?
- Which organism is most commonly implicated?
- Can you list some risk factors for septic arthritis?

REACTIVE ARTHRITIS/REITER'S SYNDROME

Reactive arthritis is a sterile arthritis occurring following an infection at a distant site. Reiter's syndrome is the triad of arthritis, urethritis and conjunctivitis.

EPIDEMIOLOGY

- Enteric source reactive arthritis has an equal sex distribution, but Reiter's syndrome is 10-20 times more common in males
- The peak age of onset is between 20 and 40
- It is more common in Caucasians
- Associated with HLA-B27

PATIENT ASSESSMENT

- Reactive arthritis tends to occur 2-4 weeks after the infection, and can last several months
- Classically there is an asymmetrical oligoarthritis of the lower limbs
- Enthesitis is common
- Dactylitis is also common
- Patients may have symptoms of urethritis

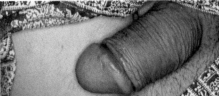

Keratoderma blennorrhagica and circinate balanitis

Photographs courtesy of the CDC/ Susan Lindsley, VD

ADDITIONAL FEATURES

- Malaise, fatigue and fever
- Up to 50% complain of lower back pain
- Conjunctivitis or anterior uveitis
- Circinate balanitis (painless inflammation of the glans penis)
- Keratoderma blennorrhagica (waxy brownish papules or scaly lesions on palms and soles)
- Oral ulcers
- Nail dystrophy
- Mild nephropathy may also occur

INVESTIGATIONS

- Inflammatory markers are usually significantly elevated
- Rheumatoid factor and ANA are negative
- Joint aspirate does not show crystals or organisms, but white cells and bacterial antigens may be present
- Stool, throat and urethral cultures are often negative by the time the arthritis has developed
- Serology for chlamydia
- X-rays are often normal acutely, but in chronic cases may show marginal erosions, particularly at the MTP joints, plantar spurs, sacroiliitis and asymmetrical syndesmophytes

MANAGEMENT BASICS

- Initially rest the joints, then physiotherapy
- NSAIDs
- Intra-articular steroids
- Antibiotics if a causative organism is found, but whether this alters the course of the arthritis is debatable
- DMARDs, particularly sulfasalazine or methotrexate should be considered for chronic or recurrent symptoms

- 10% of patients do not have a preceding symptomatic infection, 25% have recurrent episodes and 15% develop chronic arthritis

SELF ASSESSMENT

A 30 year old gentleman has a swollen left knee and right ankle. He has never had joint problems before. He returned from holiday three weeks ago, which was spoilt by a bout of diarrhoea. You suspect reactive arthritis
- Reactive arthritis is associated with which HLA antigen?
- Why should you check the soles of his feet?
- Is an intra-articular steroid injection safe?

BEHCET'S DISEASE

Behçet's disease is a complex multi-system inflammatory vasculitis characterised by oral and genital ulceration.

EPIDEMIOLOGY

- Tends to affect young adults (usually in their 30's)
- Most common along the 'silk road' from Turkey to Japan
- Gender distribution varies by region, but overall is more common and severe in men
- Associated with HLA B51, and around 30% of patients have a positive family history

PATIENT ASSESSMENT

The key features are
- Recurrent oral aphthous ulcers
- Genital ulcers
- Recurrent anterior uveitis (or other ocular involvement)
- Skin lesions or vasculitis, particularly erythema nodosum like lesions, deep vein thrombosis, thrombophlebitis, acne like lesions and pathergy reactions

ADDITIONAL FEATURES

- Constitutional symptoms: Fatigue, weight loss, generalised weakness, temperature change and lymphadenopathy
- Musculoskeletal: Arthritis which is usually asymmetrical, non erosive and predominantly affecting the lower limbs
- Neurological: Headaches, cognitive decline, aseptic meningitis, ataxia and 'brain stem syndrome'
- Gastrointestinal: Abdominal discomfort, flatulence, bloating, vomiting, diarrhoea and gastrointestinal bleeding. The ileocaecal region is the most commonly affected area
- Others: Epididymitis and arterial aneurysms

PATHERGY TESTING

- Pathergy is the only specific feature of Behçet's disease
- In a positive test, red papules appear at the site of sterile needle pricks after 48 hours
- The test is positive in over 60% of Middle Eastern patients
- However, the diagnostic value is limited in Caucasians, as it is positive in just 5%

INVESTIGATIONS

- Routine blood tests may reveal a mild anaemia and leukocytosis
- Inflammatory markers are a poor predictor of disease activity, but may be elevated.
- Immunoglobulins (especially IgA) may be elevated
- 20-30% are positive for antiphospholipid antibodies, which are associated with an increased incidence of thrombosis
- ANA and rheumatoid factor are usually negative, but p-ANCA is occasionally positive
- Pathergy testing
- Synovial fluid is often cloudy with white blood cells
- Brain imaging or angiography may be indicated

MANAGEMENT BASICS

- Patient education
- Tetracyclines are the drug of choice for oral ulcers (dissolved in water and held in the mouth for 2 minutes)
- Immunosuppression with steroids remains the mainstay of treatment
- Azathioprine, pentoxifylline, dapsone and colchicine have all been shown to have beneficial effects
- There is growing evidence for the use of anti-TNF therapy
- Additionally, sulfasalazine or mesalamine can be useful for gastrointestinal lesions, as can cyclophosphamide for vasculitis or pulmonary arterial aneurysms
- Thalidomide can be useful for treating severe ulceration
- Surgery may be required for complications

PROGNOSIS

- Onset in those younger than 25 is associated with eye involvement and more severe disease

SELF ASSESSMENT

- Name the classical triad of symptoms.
- What neurological symptoms may occur?

ANTIPHOSPHOLIPID SYNDROME

Antiphospholipid syndrome (APS) is a multi-system autoimmune disorder characterised by arterial and venous thrombosis, recurrent foetal loss and thrombocytopenia.

EPIDEMIOLOGY

- Tends to affect women of childbearing age
- There is a female:male ratio of 3.5:1 for primary APS and 7:1 for secondary APS
- APS is a major cause of strokes in young adults and of recurrent miscarriages
- May be primary or secondary, most commonly to SLE. Around one-third of patients with SLE also have APS
- Other secondary causes of APS include other autoimmune conditions, some infections and certain medications

PATIENT ASSESSMENT

- It is important to consider multiple systems and to also examine the patient for signs of a secondary cause
- The key features can be remembered using the mnemonic 'CLOT'
- Clot; arterial or venous thrombosis, such as stroke, transient ischaemic attack (TIA), pulmonary embolism and deep vein thrombosis (DVT)
- Livedo reticularis; cutaneous cyanotic vascularity
- Obstetric loss, which can occur at any gestation
- Thrombocytopenia and prolonged APTT

ADDITIONAL FEATURES

- Signs of SLE (e.g. malar rash, vasculitis or photosensitivity)
- Myocardial infarction and valvular heart disease including Libman-Sacks endocarditis
- Leg ulcers
- Raynaud's phenomenon
- Thrombosis may lead to Budd-Chiari syndrome or Addison's disease depending upon the location
- Nephropathy, renal infarction or renal vein thrombosis
- Nonthrombotic neurological symptoms can also occur, such as headaches (especially migraines), chorea, seizures and transverse myelitis
- Pulmonary hypertension
- Pre-eclampsia
- Intrauterine growth restriction

INVESTIGATIONS

- Routine blood tests including a clotting screen (thrombocytopenia, haemolytic anaemia and prolonged APTT are common)
- The Sydney criteria requires a positive lupus anticoagulant, anticardiolipin antibody or anti-beta 2 glycoprotein I on two occasions at least 12 weeks apart (and at least 12 weeks after a thrombotic event)
- Investigations relevant to presentation, such as a doppler ultrasound for suspected DVT
- ANA is less frequently positive than in SLE, but a biologic false positive serological test for syphilis is common

MANAGEMENT BASICS

- Patient education
- Lifestyle advice to reduce cardiovascular risk such as smoking cessation and regular exercise
- Management of any acute presentation
- Management of any secondary cause
- After a thrombotic event patients should be warfarinised

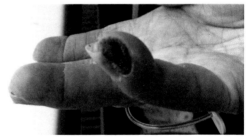

Finger necrosis in a patient with APS

- Heparin and low dose aspirin are used in pregnancy in place of warfarin

SELF ASSESSMENT

- What does the mnemonic CLOT stand for?
- If APS is a prothrombotic condition, why is there a rise in the APTT?

POLYMYALGIA RHEUMATICA

Polymyalgia rheumatica (PMR) is an inflammatory condition characterised by proximal myalgia and morning stiffness of the shoulder and hip girdles.

EPIDEMIOLOGY

- The median age of onset is 72 and it is very rare in those aged under 50
- It is most common in Northern Europeans, although it can occur in all ethnic groups
- There is a female:male ratio of 2:1
- Around 15% of patients develop giant cell arteritis, whilst 50% of patients with giant cell arteritis will have associated PMR

PATIENT ASSESSMENT

Musculoskeletal features include
- Myalgia of the shoulder and hip girdles
- The shoulders are usually affected first
- It is the muscles rather than joints that are tender
- Morning stiffness lasting longer than an hour
- Normal muscle strength
- Mild transient synovitis can occur (usually in the knees and wrists and is asymmetrical)
- In the late stages generalised muscle atrophy can occur

INVESTIGATIONS

- Anaemia of chronic disease may occur
- inflammatory markers are elevated
- Thyroid function tests (hypothyroidism is commonly associated with PMR)
- LFTs often show a raised ALP and gamma glutamyl transpeptidase (GGT)

Diagnosis of PMR is to a certain extent a diagnosis of exclusion
- ANA and rheumatoid factor (are usually negative) to differentiate PMR from connective tissue diseases
- Creatine kinase level (usually normal) to differentiate PMR from polymyositis
- Bone profile and vitamin D level to differentiate PMR from osteomalacia
- Protein electrophoresis to differentiate PMR from multiple myeloma
- Joint x-rays to exclude osteoarthritis if patient assessment is inconclusive
- Ultrasound of the shoulders may show bursitis and biceps tendon tenosynovitis and can help differentiate PMR from rotator cuff pathology

ADDITIONAL FEATURES

- Systemic features such as weight loss, fever, fatigue and lethargy
- Depression secondary to the effect on everyday life, especially if untreated
- Carpel tunnel syndrome
- Distal oedema

MANAGEMENT BASICS

- Steroids are the only effective treatment
- A typical starting dose of prednisolone would be 15mg
- The response to treatment is often dramatic and occurs within 48 hours. If it is not, the diagnosis should be reconsidered
- It is a typical aim to reduce the prednisolone to 10mg over the first 2 months and then by a further 1mg every two months thereafter (according to symptoms rather than ESR)
- Some patients require a small dose of steroid for several years
- Bone protection, usually a bisphosphonate (but at least calcium and vitamin D supplementation) should be started at the same time as the steroids
- Gastric protection is also often required

- Relapses are common as the steroids are being reduced
- The overall prognosis is excellent

SELF ASSESSMENT

A 76 year old lady presents with a two week history of aches and stiffness in the shoulder region, a low grade fever and lethargy. Baseline blood tests show an elevated ESR and ALP.
- How many differential diagnoses can you think of?
- After further assessment and investigations you diagnose polymyalgia rheumatica. What two drugs should you prescribe?
- How long would you expect her to be on this treatment?

FIBROMYALGIA

Fibromyalgia is a chronic pain disorder with multiple other symptoms and the absence of any demonstrable pathology.

EPIDEMIOLOGY

- Fibromyalgia has an estimated prevalence of around 5%
- The female:male ratio is 9:1
- The peak age of onset is between 25 and 50

PATIENT ASSESSMENT

- Diagnosis is based on the presence of widespread body pain, with no objective cause and tenderness in at least 11 of the 18 defined test points
- Other common symptoms include headaches, fatigue, sleep problems, poor cognition, non-dermatomal numbness and morning stiffness
- Additionally, patients will often complain of subjective weakness and that their joints 'feel' swollen without any objective evidence
- Fibromyalgia is still generally considered to be a diagnosis of exclusion

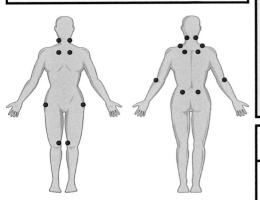

The location of the 18 test points

ADDITIONAL FEATURES

- Depression and anxiety
- Irritable bowel syndrome
- Irritable bladder
- Restless leg (Ekbom) syndrome
- Allergic or hypersensitivity symptoms
- Dysmenorrhoea or premenstrual syndrome
- Non cardiac chest pain
- Raynaud's phenomenon

INVESTIGATIONS

- Routine baseline blood tests including inflammatory markers, creatine kinase, bone profile, glucose and thyroid function tests are all likely to be normal
- An immunology screen may be ordered but one should consider the implication of false positives
- Urinalysis for blood, protein and glucose

MANAGEMENT BASICS

- Patient education and management tailored to the individual is important
- Care should be taken not to over-investigate the patient
- Exercise programmes and balneotherapy (heated pool treatment)
- Cognitive behavioural therapy and relaxation
- Tramadol is recommended for pain
- Other simple analgesics can be considered, but strong opioids and steroids should be avoided
- Antidepressants such as amitriptyline, fluoxetine and duloxetine can reduce pain and improve function
- Pramipexole and pregabalin may also have a beneficial effect on pain in some individuals
- Acupuncture or trigger point injections are not considered to be helpful

- It is estimated that at least 25% of patients with rheumatoid arthritis and 50% with SLE also have fibromyalgia

SELF ASSESSMENT

You review a 40 year old lady. She complains about pain all over her body. Examination is unremarkable apart from a number of tender points. You therefore suspect a diagnosis of fibromyalgia

- What abnormalities would you expect on her immunology screen?
- How likely is she to have joint swelling?
- She asks about a course of steroids. What would you advise?

VASCULITIS

Vasculitis is inflammation of the walls of blood vessels. This may be primary or secondary. Vasculitides are usually classified by the main type of vessel affected.

EPIDEMIOLOGY

- Vasculitis is rare with an annual incidence of 3,000 in the UK
- It can occur in childhood; Henoch-Schönlein purpura (HSP) and Kawasaki disease are the most common types
- Infections, abscesses, connective tissue disorders, malignancy and drugs are common secondary causes. However, just under half of all cases are idiopathic

RASH AND ARTHRITIS

- Vasculitis
- Infections, for example those caused by streptococcal or neisserial species, viruses or lyme disease
- Sarcoidosis (erythema nodosum)
- Connective tissue diseases
- Drug reactions
- Psoriasis

CLASSIFICATION

Small vessel vasculitis
- Allergic or hypersensitivity vasculitis
- Drug, infection or malignancy induced vasculitis
- Henoch-Schönlein purpura (HSP)
- Vasculitis of connective tissue diseases
- Cryoglobulinaemia
- Microscopic polyangiitis
Medium vessel vasculitis
- Polyarteritis nodosa
- Wegener's granulomatosis
- Churg-Strauss syndrome
- Kawasaki disease
Large vessel vasculitis
- Takayasu arteritis
- Giant cell arteritis (temporal arteritis)
- Ankylosing spondylitis associated vasculitis
Others
- Behçet's disease (vasculitis and venulitis)

PATIENT ASSESSMENT

- The history should include questions about potential secondary causes and constitutional symptoms such as fever, night sweats, malaise and weight loss
- The rash itself may be purpuric, maculopapular or livedo reticularis

ADDITIONAL FEATURES

- Musculoskeletal: Arthralgia or arthritis
- Renal: Glomerulonephritis
- Neurological: Mononeuritis multiplex
- Respiratory: Dyspnoea, haemoptysis or cough
- Cardiovascular: Pericarditis or myocarditis
- Gastrointestinal: Pain, diarrhoea or bleeding secondary to ulceration
- Ocular: Retinal haemorrhage

HENOCH-SCHONLEIN PURPURA

- Tends to affect children aged 3-10 years
- Characterised by IgA deposition
- Acute presentations often occur in the winter months (post upper respiratory tract infection) and are usually self limiting
- Purpuric rash (especially over the legs and buttocks), abdominal pain, nephritis and arthritis are the key features
- As HSP is usually self limiting it does not require specific treatment
- The initial episode can last several months and one third have future reoccurrences

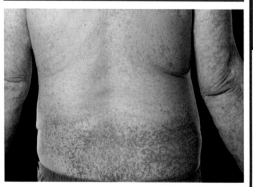

A gentleman with a vasculitic rash secondary to Henoch-Schönlein purpura

VASCULITIS

INVESTIGATIONS

- Routine blood tests may show a normochromic normocytic anaemia, neutrophilia and raised inflammatory markers
- Eosinophilia can occur in any vasculitis but is most characteristic of Churg-Strauss syndrome
- Anti-neutrophil cytoplasmic antibodies (ANCA). A cytoplasmic staining pattern (cANCA) is associated with Wegener's granulomatosis. A perinuclear staining pattern (pANCA) is associated with Churg-Strauss syndrome and microscopic polyangiitis
- Rheumatoid factor is frequently positive
- An ANA is useful, as a positive result is suggestive of a secondary connective tissue disorder
- Cryoglobulins
- Urinalysis for protein, blood and glucose
- Urine protein:creatinine ratio
- A chest x-ray may show diffuse or nodular shadowing
- Biopsies as appropriate
- Arteriography in polyarteritis nodosa looking for multiple small aneurysms

WEGENER'S GRANULOMATOSIS

- A rare granulomatous necrotising vasculitis
- Can affect any organ, but there is a classical triad of sinusitis type symptoms, respiratory problems and renal involvment
- cANCA is positive in around 90%
- Untreated Wegener's granulomatosis has a very poor prognosis

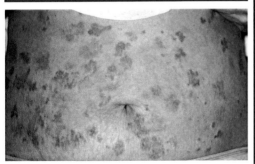

A lady with vasculitic lesions secondary to Systemic lupus erythematosus. Note that the lesions are of various ages

POLYARTERITIS NODOSA

- A necrotising vasculitis of small to medium sized vessels
- Most common in middle aged men and is associated with hepatitis B infection
- Skin, renal, neurological, cardiovascular, gastrointestinal and musculoskeletal systems are frequently involved
- Renal failure can be rapid
- Microaneurysms are characteristic
- A more limited form has also been described; cutaneous polyarteritis nodosa (CPAN)

MANAGEMENT BASICS

- Remove or treat any precipitating factors or conditions (around 50% of patients presenting with vasculitis will have a treatable cause)
- Steroids are the mainstay of treatment
- Immunosuppressive agents (such as cyclophosphamide and azathioprine) for medium vessel and a few small or large vessel vasculitides
- There is likely to be a growth in the use of biological agents
- In fulminant cases plasma exchange and immunoglobulins should be considered
- A key exception to the above is Kawasaki disease in which steroids are contraindicated. Instead aspirin and in some cases intravenous immunoglobulins is the main treatment

CHURG-STRAUSS SYNDROME

- A rare diffuse vasculitis affecting small to medium sized vessels
- Classically associated with asthma and eosinophilia
- Mononeuritis multiplex is common
- There tends to be three phases of presentation; prodromal symptoms of asthma or rhinitis, eosinophilic pneumonia or gastritis and then systemic vasculitis
- pANCA is positive in around 70% of patients
- There is evidence that leukotriene receptor antagonists used in the treatment of asthma may precipitate the condition

VASCULITIS

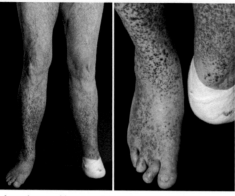

A gentleman with a vasculitic rash and amputation

TAKAYASU ARTERITIS

- Is commonly known as the 'pulseless disease' as the effect on the aorta and main branches produces absent pulses as well as arm claudication and bruits
- Most commonly affects young females, particularly in Asia and Japan
- Systemic illness, hypertension and visual disturbance is common
- More serious complications include stroke and myocardial infarction
- Diagnosis is confirmed by imaging

GIANT CELL ARTERITIS

- Giant cell (or temporal) arteritis occurs almost exclusively in the over 50's, but is relatively common
- It affects women two to three times more commonly than men
- There is a close clinical relationship with polymyalgia rheumatica
- Classically there is a temporal headache with tender, enlarged, non-pulsatile temporal arteries
- Patients also frequently complain of pain brushing their hair (scalp tenderness) and jaw claudication whilst masticating
- Systemic symptoms such as fever, malaise, fatigue and weight loss can occur
- Visual disturbance (such as blurred vision or diplopia) occurs in around 50% of cases and can precede the headache
- Visual loss can occur secondary to ischaemic optic neuropathy
- High dose prednisolone must be started early to prevent visual loss which is often permanent
- If visual loss is a presenting feature, the patient should see an ophthalmologist the same day
- ESR is typically elevated
- Temporal artery biopsy (be aware that skip lesions can occur) is the diagnostic investigation of choice
- If there is not a dramatic improvement with high dose prednisolone the diagnosis should be reconsidered
- Aortitis and aortic aneurysm or dissection are important complications
- Renal involvement is rare

- Regular monitoring of renal function and urinalysis is vital as renal involvement of vasculitis is a key determinant of prognosis
- Certain mimics of vasculitis should be excluded, such as subacute endocarditis, atrial myxoma, thrombotic thrombocytopenic purpura and cholesterol embolism

SELF ASSESSMENT

For each of the below, which type of vasculitis is most likely?

- A 41 year old man with asthma, eosinophilia and mononeuritis multiplex.
- A 41 year old man with chronic sinusitis and a saddle shaped nose.
- A 29 year old IV drug user who is hepatitis C positive.
- A 21 year old Japanese lady with a significant blood pressure difference between her arms.
- A 41 year old man with a positive p-ANCA, hepatitis B and microaneurysms in the small and medium sized arteries of his kidneys.
- A 9 year old girl with joint pains and a purpuric rash mainly over her buttocks.
- A 77 year old man with scalp tenderness and myalgia around his shoulders and hips.
- A 1 year old boy with inflammation of his lips and tongue and bilateral conjunctivitis.

It's Friday afternoon and you see a 69 year old man with a two week unilateral headache and visual disturbance for two days. You suspect temporal arteritis.

- What are the two most important management steps?
- In temporal arteritis what should you be able to feel when you palpate for a temporal artery pulse?

JUVENILE IDIOPATHIC ARTHRITIS

Juvenile idiopathic arthritis (JIA) is a group of heterogeneous disease subtypes characterised by arthritis of unknown aetiology occurring before the age of 16 and lasting for more than 6 weeks.

EPIDEMIOLOGY

- The prevalence of JIA is around 0.1-0.2%
- The oligoarticular and polyarticular forms are more common in girls, whilst the systemic form has an equal gender distribution

PATIENT ASSESSMENT

- The clinical presentation of JIA often varies
- A child's age and developmental stage will impact upon how they communicate their joint pain and dysfunction
- Pain tends to be a mild to moderate ache that is worse on movement
- Morning stiffness can occur and parents may describe their child as 'slow to get going'
- Large joints are more frequently affected, although small joints are affected in polyarticular disease
- On examination, joints can be warm and swollen, but are not usually erythematous
- The temporomandibular joint and spine should not be neglected on examination
- The extra-articular features listed below are rare in the oligoarticular form

ADDITIONAL FEATURES

- Uveitis
- Fever, fatigue and weight loss
- Rash (classically salmon-pink macules)
- Hepatosplenomegaly and lymphadenopathy
- Pleuritis, pericarditis, peritonitis and myocarditis may occur
- Complications including osteoporosis, generalised growth restriction, medication side effects and psychosocial, behavioural and educational problems

INVESTIGATIONS

- The diagnosis of JIA is largely clinical
- Inflammatory markers may be raised and there may be anaemia of chronic disease
- ANA positivity confers an increased risk of developing uveitis and rheumatoid factor has prognostic significance
- Joint imaging can help confirm the diagnosis and exclude differential diagnoses

ILAR CLASSIFICATION

1. Systemic arthritis (10-20%)
- Fever of at least two weeks in duration (and quotidian in nature for at least three days) and at least one of the following:
    - Transient salmon coloured rash
    - Generalized lymphadenopathy
    - Hepatomegaly or splenomegaly
    - Serositis
2. Oligoarthritis (50-60%)
- Four or less joints affected in the first six months
- If more joints become involved later the term 'extended' is used
3. Polyarthritis (25-35%)
- Five or more joints affected in the first six months
- Can be further divided into rheumatoid factor positive or negative
4. Psoriatic arthritis (5-15%)
- Arthritis with psoriasis
- Or arthritis with two of dactylitis, nail pitting or onycholysis and psoriasis in a first degree relative
5. Enthesitis related arthritis (1-7%)
- Arthritis and enthesitis
- Or arthritis or enthesitis with at least two of
    - HLA-B27 positive sacroiliac or inflammatory lumbar spine pain
    - Onset in a male aged over 6 years
    - Acute (symptomatic) anterior uveitis
    - Relevant family history
6. Undifferentiated arthritis
- Arthritis that fulfils none or more than one of the above criteria

MANAGEMENT BASICS

- Treatment aims are to prevent joint pain and damage and to preserve normal development
- The main drug treatments are NSAIDs, DMARDs and biological agents
- Methotrexate is well tolerated and is the most frequently used DMARD, and adalimumab and etanercept have a licence for use in JIA
- The use of steroids is minimised despite their effectiveness due to their side effects
- Physiotherapy, occupational therapy and liaison with schools is important
- Ophthalmic opinion if uveitis occurs

IMMUNOLOGY OVERVIEW

RHEUMATOID FACTOR

- An IgM antibody which reacts with the Fc portion of human IgG
- It is positive in 70% of patients with rheumatoid arthritis and higher titres are associated with more severe disease
- 5% of the normal population are positive, however this increases to 20% in the elderly

Other conditions with a positive result

- Connective tissue disorders including Sjögren's syndrome (>95%), systemic sclerosis (30%), SLE (25%), dermatomyositis (>5%) and Felty's syndrome (>95%)
- Chronic infections including infective endocarditis (30%), pulmonary tuberculosis (10%), leprosy (50%) and syphilis (10%)
- Others include hepatitis and autoimmune liver disease, sarcoidosis, HIV, malignancy and transplant recipients

ANTI-CYCLIC CITRULLINATED PEPTIDE

- Has a similar sensitivity to rheumatoid factor (70%), but is much more specific (95%)
- It can be detectable up to 15 years prior to the development of symptoms of rheumatoid arthritis

ANTINUCLEAR ANTIBODY

- The key association is with connective tissue disorders including drug induced lupus (100%), SLE (98%), mixed connective tissue disease (95%), polymyositis/dermatomyositis (60%), systemic sclerosis (90%), Sjögren's syndrome (75%) and others
- Associations with nonrheumatic conditions include autoimmune thyroid disease, autoimmune liver diseases, some pulmonary conditions and haematological malignancies
- ANA against double stranded DNA (anti-dsDNA) is highly specific for SLE (sensitivity is 70%), but in drug induced lupus the ANA targets single stranded DNA (anti-ssDNA)

Staining patterns

- Homogeneous suggests SLE
- Nucleolar suggests systemic sclerosis
- Speckled suggests a mixed connective tissue disorder
- Centromere suggests limited systemic sclerosis (CREST)

EXTRACTABLE NUCLEAR ANTIGENS

The ENA screen is more specific for a particular condition, whereas ANA is sensitive
- Anti-Ro: Sjögren's syndrome, congenital heart block and neonatal lupus
- Anti-La: Primary Sjögren's syndrome
- Anti-Sm: SLE, particularly CNS lupus
- Anti-RNP: Mixed connective tissue disease
- Anti-Scl70: Diffuse systemic sclerosis
- Anti-centromere: Limited systemic sclerosis
- Anti-Jo1: Polymyositis (particularly lung involvement)

ANTI-NEUTROPHIL CYTOPLASMIC ANTIBODY

- Anti-neutrophil cytoplasmic antibodies are associated with vasculitis
- A cytoplasmic staining pattern (cANCA) is found in 90% of patients with Wegener's granulomatosis and in 35% of patients with microscopic polyangiitis
- Perinuclear staining pattern (pANCA) is much less specific but is associated with microscopic polyangiitis (60%), Churg-Strauss syndrome (60%), idiopathic Type III crescentic glomerulonephritis (80%), Wegener's granulomatosis (20%), some connective tissue disorders (SLE, rheumatoid arthritis and Sjögren's syndrome) and other vasculitides
- An atypical p-ANCA is associated with inflammatory bowel disease and rheumatoid arthritis

- Anticardiolipin antibodies (ACLA) are the most frequently measured antiphospholipid antibody type
- There are additional antibodies detectable in systemic sclerosis; anti-RNA-polymerases (associated with renal involvement in diffuse disease), anti-fibrillarin (U3RNP) antibody (associated with pulmonary hypertension in diffuse disease) and Anti-PM-Scl antibody (associated with the systemic sclerosis and polymyositis overlap syndrome)
- Anti-histone antibodies are associated with drug induced lupus
- Anti-Mi2 antibodies are associated with dermatomyositis

DMARDS – THE MAIN FIVE

DMARDs (disease modifying anti-rheumatic drugs) are used to halt disease progression. Regular monitoring of blood tests and for clinical signs and symptoms of toxicity is essential.

METHOTREXATE

- A dihydrofolate reductase which tends to be first line in the management of rheumatoid arthritis
- Oral administration is preferred, although it can be given subcutaneously if side effects are a problem (the intramuscular route may also be considered)
- A typical dose is 7.5-25mg weekly
- It is usually co-prescribed with folic acid, as this reduces the toxic side effects and therefore improves compliance
- Response time is 6-12 weeks
- Trimethoprim or co-trimoxazole should not be prescribed with methotrexate due to the increased risk of bone marrow aplasia
- Some sources will state that caution should be taken with NSAIDs and penicillins as methotrexate is renally excreted, but clinically significant interactions are rare
- Methotrexate has the potential to cause hepatotoxicity and pulmonary toxicity and is teratogenic. Therefore advice about alcohol and contraception is extremely important

LEFLUNOMIDE

- Is a relatively new DMARD which inhibits the de novo synthesis of pyrimidines by inhibiting dihydroorotate dehydrogenase which then has a knock on effect on lymphocytes
- It is given orally, with a typical dose of 10-20mg
- It has a very long half life and therefore loading doses of 100mg can be used. This is now much less common in practice due to side effects (particularly diarrhoea)
- Response time is 8-12 weeks (or longer without a loading dose)
- Leflunomide is teratogenic and due to its long half life women are advised not to conceive within 2 years of stopping treatment. Men are are advised to use contraception for 3 months after stopping
- Live vaccines should be avoided
- There is a 10% risk of hypertension and so monitoring of blood pressure is important
- Due to the long half life, when serious side effects occur a washout with cholestyramine or activated charcoal for 11 days is needed. This is unpleasant and may put some off using the drug

SULFASALAZINE

- Is a combination of an antibacterial agent (sulfapyridine) and an anti-inflammatory agent (5-aminosalicylic acid)
- It is given orally and a typical dose would be 500mg increased weekly to between 2-3 grams a day (in 2-3 divided doses)
- Response time is around 12 weeks
- It may cause drug induced lupus in slow acetylators
- It can also cause a reduction of sperm counts in men
- It should not be prescribed to patients who have an allergy to aspirin or sulfa containing drugs

AZATHIOPRINE

- Is a prodrug of mercaptopurine having both cytotoxic and immunosuppressive effects
- It is usually given orally (the intravenous route is very irritant) and a typical starting dose would be 1mg/kg/day. This can be increased to 2-3mg/kg/day after 4-6 weeks
- Response time is 6-12 weeks
- All patients should have their thiopurine methyl transferase (TPMT) level checked. Deficiency (heterozygous state) is associated with serious (even fatal) toxicity. Higher levels indicate the need for higher doses
- If co-prescribed with allopurinol the dose should be reduced by 25%
- It can inhibit the anti-coagulant effect of warfarin and can cause anaemia in combination with an ACE inhibitor
- Live vaccines should be avoided

HYDROXYCHLOROQUINE

- An antimalarial often used in SLE and rheumatoid arthritis
- With rheumatoid arthritis, evidence for joint protection is limited and so combination with another DMARD is common
- It is administered orally at a dose of between 200-400mg a day
- It may be safe in pregnancy, although data is limited
- Patients should be advised to report any visual problems due to the risk of retinopathy

BIOLOGICAL THERAPIES

TUMOUR NECROSIS FACTOR (TNF)

• Is a key proinflammatory cytokine released by macrophages
• Levels have been found to be elevated in the serum and synovium of patients with rheumatoid arthritis
• It signals for inflammatory molecules and directly stimulates neutrophils and fibroblasts to produce a variety of enzymes which damage joints
• This has lead to the rise of anti-TNF therapy

ANTI-TNF AGENTS

Infliximab (Remicade)
• A chimeric (human and murine) monoclonal antibody
• Given intravenously over 4 hours every 4-8 weeks
• Has a higher immunogenicity than other anti-TNF therapies and so methotrexate is often used concurrently to prevent neutralising antibody formation.
Etanercept (Enbrel)
• A fully human dimeric, soluble, fusion protein
• Administered subcutaneously two times a week
• Has a licence for use in children
Adalimumab (Humira)
• A fully human recombinant monoclonal antibody
• Administered subcutaneously every two weeks
Others
• Newer agents include certolizumab (Cimzia) and golimumab (Simponi)

RISKS ASSOCIATED WITH ANTI-TNF AGENTS

• Risk of severe infections, most notably tuberculosis (TNF is required for granuloma formation and maintenance)
• Although there is probably no increased risk of overall malignancy, concern remains over non melanoma skin cancers
• Demyelination
• Worsening of cardiac failure

ANTI-TNF ASSESSMENT

• The British Society for Rheumatology (BSR) and NICE recommend that to commence on anti-TNF therapy patients must have severe rheumatoid arthritis (a DAS28 score over 5.1 on two occasions at least a month apart)
• Patients should also have failed at least two DMARDs
• Patients must be screened for tuberculosis and hepatitis
• Cautions and contraindications include significant liver and renal impairment, cardiac failure, demyelination, septic arthritis in the last 12 months, pregnancy and breast feeding
• Patients should be advised to avoid live vaccines whilst having anti-TNF therapy

RITUXIMAB

• A chimeric (human and murine) monoclonal antibody
• Targets B lymphocytes displaying the CD20 cell surface marker
• Two intravenous infusions are administered two weeks apart
• Maximal benefit is achieved after 16 weeks
• Infusion reactions are relatively common
• Due to the success of rituximab, other B cell depleting drugs are being developed and evaluated targeting either CD20 or CD22

• Is a fusion protein that inhibits the co-stimulation of T cells ultimately leading to reduced cytokine production
• Administered as an intravenous infusion
• At present has not been approved by NICE

TOCILIZUMAB

• An interleukin-6 receptor antagonist
• Administered by intravenous infusion over an hour every 4 weeks
• NICE recommend its use when a patient has failed at least one anti-TNF therapy and rituximab (or there was an adverse reaction to these drugs or they are contraindicated)
• Usually given with methotrexate
• A subcutaneous form is currently being evaluated

ANSWERS

RHEUMATOID ARTHRITIS

You order blood tests, what is the probability that she is rheumatoid factor positive?

70-80% of patients with rheumatoid arthritis are rheumatoid factor positive. However, 5% of the normal population are also positive.

You have obtained baseline blood test results, give an example of an appropriate drug regime?

In keeping with the 2009 NICE guidelines, methotrexate, sulfasalazine and a short course of prednisolone would be most appropriate and should be started as soon as possible after the diagnosis is made. Analgesia should be offered; paracetamol and codeine are first line. It is also important not to forget about contraception in the relevant group of patients (that would include this lady).

Six months later, she develops a red eye. There is no pain or itch and her vision is normal. What is the most likely cause?

There are a few key points to remember. Keratoconjunctivitis sicca is the most common eye problem amongst patients with rheumatoid arthritis. In terms of a red eye, episcleritis is painless and scleritis is painful. Corneal ulceration, keratitis, steroid induced cataracts and retinopathy secondary to hydroxychloroquine can also occur. Therefore this patient most likely has episcleritis.

At the same review, you note that she is anaemic. Can you list any potential explanations?

Anaemia of chronic disease

Iron deficiency anaemia, especially if taking NSAIDs (due to gastric blood loss)

Haemolytic (which can be secondary to sulfasalazine)

Secondary to methotrexate

Secondary to rare associated features such as Felty syndrome

Aplastic (rare)

At a later review she complains that she is finding it difficult to chew and swallow food. What else should you ask her and what is the most likely explanation?

You should ask her about dry eyes and if appropriate organise a Schirmer lacrimation test as these symptoms could well represent Sjögren's syndrome.

You also order hand x-rays, what changes will you be looking for?

Loss of joint space, peri-articular osteopenia, bony erosions, soft tissue swelling and subluxation, particularly at the MCP joints. You should also have requested x-rays of the feet.

SLE

What other symptoms should you ask about?

These are multiple, but should include systemic symptoms, other rashes, general and specific aches and pains elsewhere, mucosal ulcers, alopecia, headaches (particularly migraines), seizures, depression, dry mouth or eyes, any other eye problem and the symptoms of secondary antiphospholipid syndrome (such as miscarriages, leg ulcers and previous deep vein thrombosis).

Which blood tests should you request?

Routine blood tests (FBC, U&Es, LFTs), inflammatory markers (ESR and CRP), clotting screen (due to the prolonged APTT in antiphospholipid syndrome), ANA, ENA, dsDNA antibodies, complement levels, immunoglobulins and plasma electrophoresis. Anticardiolipin antibodies and lupus anticoagulant may be requested if indicated.

If her ANA comes back as negative, could she still have SLE?

98% of patients with SLE are ANA positive, which of course means that 2% are negative. However most of these remaining 2% are ENA positive, so if a patient is both ANA and ENA negative, SLE is unlikely.

What haematological abnormalities might be seen in a patient with SLE?

It is easy to remember as everything goes down; anaemia, leucopenia, lymphopenia and thrombocytopenia. It is worth bearing in mind that some treatments might have similar effects.

In fact her ANA, dsDNA antibodies and anti-sm antibodies are all positive and this confirms the diagnosis of SLE. What advice would you give her about triggers of disease activity?

Triggers of flares of SLE include overexposure to sunlight, infections, stress and oestrogen containing medications. Therefore advice should include sun avoidance and use of sunscreens, recognising when they feel unwell, taking time to relax and avoiding certain oral contraceptive pills (and discussing other forms of contraception if necessary). Other general lifestyle advice about diet, not smoking and exercise is encouraged.

Which blood tests can be used to monitor disease activity in this patient?

Complement levels (go down), dsDNA (goes up, and can only be used if the patient is initially positive), ESR (goes up). CRP classically does not increase during a flare of SLE and if raised should raise the possibility of infection, however the small print reads that it can increase with active serositis or arthritis.

ANSWERS

What is the most commonly affected organ in SLE and what therefore must you do at every follow up appointment?

The kidneys. Every patient requires a blood pressure measurement (checking for hypertension), and a urine dipstick (checking for protein and blood).

If you performed hand x-rays on this lady, what type of erosions might you see?

Classically the arthritis associated with SLE is non-erosive, however deformities can still occur.

Which organs are classically spared?

The kidneys and brain.

What is the key management step?

Stop the offending drug, in this case, minocycline.

PSORIATIC ARTHRITIS

What percentage of patients with psoriasis go on to develop associated arthropathy?

10%

What are the key features from the history, examination and investigations that would point you towards a diagnosis of psoriatic rather than coincidental rheumatoid arthritis?

The key distinguishing features are the presence of nail changes (PsA), DIP joint involvement (PsA), dactylitis (PsA), nodules (RA), hand deformity (usually worse in RA), systemic features (more common in RA), rheumatoid factor and anti-CCP antibodies (not diagnostic either way) and x-ray changes (such as peri-articular osteopenia).

In the context of psoriatic arthritis, can you explain the ankle pain?

Enthesitis of the Achilles tendon.

Whilst the management of psoriatic arthritis is similar to that of rheumatoid arthritis, some medications can lead to a flare of the skin disease. Can you name some?

NSAIDs and hydroxychloroquine. With oral steroids there may be a rebound worsening of the skin when the steroids are stopped.

What is the 'pencil in cup' deformity and which other characteristic x-ray changes can you list?

A pencil in cup deformity is where the distal end of a bone becomes pointed as can be seen at some of the PIP joints on the x-ray on page 8. Other x-ray changes include para-marginal erosions, asymmetrical sacroiliitis, unilateral spinal syndesmophytes and fluffy periosteal bone formation.

In a patient without known psoriasis, in which 'hidden' areas should you check?

The hairline, particularly behind the ears, the umbilicus and in the natal cleft.

GOUT

What is the main causative factor of gout?

90% of cases of gout are due to under-excretion of uric acid.

You examine his hands but can't see any tophi. Where else should you specifically look? Why might you not see any in this patient?

Feet, elbows and the pinna of the ear. Tophi can also be found on tendons elsewhere. Tophi are classically seen in cases of chronic gout.

If this was pseudogout, what might you see on his x-ray?

Chondrocalcinosis.

You aspirate his joint, and on microscopy you see needle shaped crystals and no organisms. Given the diagnosis, what would be the most appropriate initial therapy? What is the main side effect?

Colchicine and diarrhoea.

NSAIDs should be avoided due to his renal failure. Steroids (especially oral) are likely to upset his glycaemic control. An intra-articular joint injection would be less problematic but in this patient most would favour colchicine, which is safe in renal failure as long as creatinine clearance is above 10ml/min.

Why might his urate level be normal?

Urate levels often fall during an acute attack of gout. This is why its diagnostic value is limited.

Which joint would have been more classical for a first presentation?

The 1st metatarsophalangeal joint is affected in 70% of first and 50% of all presentations.

On discharge what general advice should you give him?

Advise a sensible alcohol intake (especially beer and spirits) and to avoid dehydration.

Avoid purine rich foods (e.g. seafood and red meat), although certain purine rich vegetables are acceptable in moderation. Certain foods such as dairy products, cherries and those rich in vitamin C may be protective.

Weight reduction, regular exercise and smoking cessation are also important.

How many further attacks in the next 12 months does he need to have before you start prophylaxis, and which agent would you use?

This is a trick question. As he has renal disease he would automatically qualify for gout prophylaxis. If it wasn't for his renal disease the answer would be one, as two or more episodes in 12 months is an indication for gout prophylaxis. Allopurinol is the first line agent and is safe in renal failure.

ANSWERS

This gentleman goes on to have chronic gout, particularly affecting his hands and feet. What are the key x-ray findings you might see (or not see)?

Chronic gout classically produces 'punched out' erosions and subcortical cysts. Also bear in mind the absence of signs of other conditions; peri-articular osteopenia, osteophytes, etc.

You are asked to review a different gentleman with a raised urate level, who is asymptomatic. Should you offer him treatment?

Hyperuricaemia is relatively common and is most often asymptomatic and co-incidental. The current advice is that asymptomatic hyperuricaemia does not require treatment, however there is growing evidence that hyperuricaemia may have long term detrimental effects on health.

OSTEOPOROSIS

What lifestyle factors should you ask him about?

Questions about lifestyle should focus on his typical diet, amount of exercise, his daily or weekly alcohol intake, smoking status and sun exposure.

What key blood test should you request for a middle-aged man?

A testosterone level should always be requested in a middle aged man.

You are rightly concerned about osteoporosis. Would calcium with vitamin D supplements or a bisphosphonate be most appropriate?

It is recommended that anybody over the age of 65 who is likely to be taking more than 5mg prednisolone for at least 3 months should be prescribed a bisphosphonate (and calcium with vitamin D)

Should you perform a DEXA scan?

As this gentleman is over 65, a DEXA scan is not necessary.

Other than steroids, can you name another drug that can cause osteoporosis?

Heparin is the other key medication that you should be aware of as a cause of osteoporosis.

What does this T score mean?

A T score between −1 and −2.5 represents osteopenia.

What treatment would be most appropriate?

The T score in this patient is an indication for calcium with vitamin D and a bisphosphonate. Additionally, if her DMARDs are not controlling her rheumatoid arthritis it is worth considering her for biological therapy so that her future steroid use can be minimised.

SYSTEMIC SLEROSIS

What does CREST stand for?

CREST stands for calcinosis, Raynaud's phenomenon, oesophageal dysmotility, sclerodactyly and telangiectasia. It is a form of limited cutaneous systemic sclerosis.

Which of the five features is she most likely to have developed first?

Raynaud's phenomenon is most frequently the first symptom to develop.

Is she likely to have a better or worse prognosis than the lady with CREST?

Diffuse cutaneous limited sclerosis carries a worse prognosis than CREST (or other forms of limited disease). Male sex and Caucasian ethnicity also confer a worse prognosis.

She complains of symptoms of malabsorption. Why does this occur in systemic sclerosis?

Malabsorption can occur secondary to bacterial overgrowth.

Is she more likely to develop pulmonary hypertension or renal crisis?

Renal crisis is more common than pulmonary hypertension in those with diffuse disease. Interestingly, with the limited form it is the other way around.

What non-drug management advice could you offer her?

Firstly, the nature of the condition should be explained. Non-drug advice may include the use of makeup as camouflage and moisturising cream for dry skin, home exercises (and referral to physiotherapy), nutritional and weight loss help and guidance and the recommendation of smoking cessation as appropriate.

Why should high dose steroids be avoided in a patient with diffuse cutaneous systemic sclerosis?

High dose steroids are associated with a higher risk of developing renal crisis. This is particularly important to be aware of in patients with overlap syndromes.

How can surgery have a role in patients with systemic sclerosis?

Surgery can be used to release contractures or remove any problematic calcinosis.

Watermelon stomach is listed in the additional features section, but what is it?

Watermelon stomach is often more accurately termed gastric antral vascular ectasia (GAVE), and is therefore a type of arteriovenous malformation secondary to bleeding from the stomach. The term watermelon stomach comes from the characteristic stripes that are seen on endoscopy.

ANSWERS

RAYNAUD'S PHENOMENON

What is the difference between primary and secondary RP?

Primary RP is generally a benign condition not associated with any other disease and represents an exaggerated response to cold or emotional stimuli. It tends to begin in the teens to early 20s and has a genetic component with 30% having an affected first degree relative. Secondary RP is classified as being related to a background condition such as connective tissue disorders, peripheral vascular disease or thoracic outlet syndrome. Secondary RP often occurs in a slightly older age group, is more likely to be asymmetrical and can occur all year round.

What general advice can you give to a patient with RP?

The aim of the advice is to reduce exposure to stimuli that cause symptoms. The most important message is with regard to avoiding the cold. Smoking cessation may help reduce severity but not the occurrence of symptoms. Avoiding caffeine containing drinks and performing regular hand and feet exercises (to improve their circulation) can reduce the frequency of attacks. Other simple tips, such as avoiding carrying bags by the handles as this impairs circulation to the fingers can also make a difference . There is little objective evidence for any nutritional supplements. Minimising stress can also be effective in reducing symptoms.

Which antihypertensive should be avoided?

It is well recognised that beta blockers can exacerbate symptoms of RP, but the mechanism is still not fully understood.

SJOGREN'S SYNDROME

Which two antibodies from the ENA screen are most likely to be positive?

Anti-Ro antibodies are positive in 70% and anti-La antibodies are positive in 30% of patients with primary Sjögren's syndrome.

She has a Schirmer test. What is this?

It is a test to measure tear formation. Filter paper is placed in the lower fornix of the eye for 5 minutes and the length of paper that has become wet in that period is measured. A normal response is more than 10mm.

She continues to struggle with her dry mouth despite artificial saliva. Which medication could you try?

Pilocarpine may stimulate saliva production in this lady.

ANKYLOSING SPONDYLITIS

What is Schober's test?

Schober's test assesses the lumbar spines contribution to forward flexion. Mark lines 10cm above and 5cm below the iliac crest. When the patient bends forward, the distance between the lines should increase by more than 5cm.

Which DMARD is most frequently used in AS?

As a whole DMARDs are ineffective for disease affecting the axial skeleton. They may however have a role in controlling peripheral synovitis. Sulfasalazine is usually the drug of choice.

OSTEOARTHRITIS

What do you know of the role of glucosamine?

Some studies have shown that glucosamine can have a modest analgesic effect, especially in knee OA, but overall the evidence is mixed. Therefore the 2008 NICE guidelines do not recommend its use due to limited evidence of cost effectiveness.

In which order would you try analgesics for a lady with knee OA?

Paracetamol and topical NSAIDs are first line. Be aware that gastric side effects can still occur with topical NSAIDs. Second line would be oral NSAIDs or COX-2 inhibitors, as long as the patient is not taking aspirin. A proton pump inhibitor should be co-prescribed. If this fails to control the pain, non pharmacological measures should be re-evaluated. Opioids are the next step, although evidence suggests that low dose co-codamol does not give any additional benefit compared to paracetamol alone, and therefore higher doses of codeine should be prescribed. If the patient continues to have pain, an intra-articular steroid injection may be suitable and if the OA is impacting upon quality of life, surgical intervention should be considered. Additionally, capsaicin, a topical treatment, may be of some benefit to individuals with knee or hand OA.

PAGET'S DISEASE

What percentage of patients with Paget's disease are symptomatic at presentation?

Only 5%.

Which bones are most frequently affected?

The most frequently affected sites are the pelvis, lumbar spine, femur and skull.

What is the mainstay drug treatment?

Bisphosphonates. Analgesia is also important.

ANSWERS

POLYMYOSITIS & DERMATOMYOSITIS

What characteristic skin lesions might you see?

A photosensitive rash, a macular rash over his upper back, shoulders and chest (it classically spares the centre of the back), erythema on the extensor surface of joints, a purple heliotrope rash in the periorbital region, and Gottron's papules; roughened papules over the extensor surfaces of the fingers. There may also be nailfold capillary dilatation.

What is the likelihood that he is anti-Jo1 antibody positive?

It is unlikely as anti-Jo1 antibodies are associated with polymyositis rather than dermatomyositis.

What serious association would you want to screen him for?

You should always consider malignancy in a patient with dermatomyositis (and to a lesser extent with polymyositis). Around 25% of patients with dermatomyositis have an underlying malignancy. This risk is even higher if the patient is older.

SEPTIC ARTHRITIS

You aspirate the joint. What are the most important tests to request?

Cell counts (red and white blood cells), a gram stain, culture and microscopy (to check for crystals).

What empirical treatment does the BNF advise whilst awaiting the results?

Antibiotics that have good gram positive cover, namely flucloxacillin or clindamycin if penicillin allergic. You should however always check your local guidelines.

Which joint is most commonly affected?

The knee is affected in 50% of cases. That is if you don't count prosthetic joints!

Which organism is most commonly implicated?

Staphylococcus aureus.

Can you list some risk factors for septic arthritis?

There are a number of risk factors, but the important ones include rheumatoid arthritis, previous gout, a prosthetic joint, previous trauma, immunosuppression (which may be from treatment for a rheumatological problem), intravenous drug use, a history of sexually transmitted infections and tick bites.

REACTIVE ARTHRITIS

Reactive arthritis is associated with which HLA antigen?

HLA B27.

Why should you check the soles of his feet?

He may have the waxy yellow-brown rash of keratoderma blenorrhagica.

Would an intra-articular steroid injection be safe?

A classical feature of reactive arthritis is that no organisms can be recovered from the affected joints. White cells and bacterial antigens however may be present in the synovial fluid. As a result it is safe and usually helpful to give an intra-articular steroid injection.

BEHCET'S DISEASE

Name the classical triad of symptoms.

The classical triad of symptoms are oral aphthous ulcers, genital ulcers and anterior uveitis. Skin lesions are also very common, but pathergy is the only specific feature of Behçet's disease.

What neurological symptoms may occur?

Neurological symptoms can include headaches, cognitive decline, aseptic meningitis, ataxia and 'brain stem syndrome'.

ANTIPHOSPHOLIPID SYNDROME

What does the mnemonic CLOT stand for?

It stands for clot, livedo reticularis, obstetric loss and thrombocytopenia.

If APS is a prothrombotic condition, why is there a rise in the APTT?

This is a key point about APS, as the rise in the APTT is paradoxical given the thrombocytopenia and prothrombotic nature of the condition. However, it is due to the lupus anticoagulant autoantibodies reacting with the phospholipids in the coagulation cascade.

POLYMYALGIA RHEUMATICA

How many differential diagnoses can you think of?

Suggestions include polymyalgia rheumatica, a

ANSWERS

viral syndrome, polymyositis, dermatomyositis or other myopathy, hypothyroidism, osteomalacia, fibromyalgia or other chronic pain syndrome, depression, shoulder problems (rotator cuff pathology or adhesive capsulitis), multiple myeloma or other malignancy, connective tissue disease (such as systemic sclerosis or SLE), rheumatoid arthritis, osteoarthritis and parkinsonism.

After further assessment and investigations you diagnose polymyalgia rheumatica. What two drugs should you prescribe?

Prednisolone and a bisphosphonate such as alendronate (she is over 65 and is therefore considered a high fracture risk). Gastric protection, such as with a proton pump inhibitor and calcium with vitamin D supplementation should also be considered.

How long would you expect her to be on this treatment?

The aim should be to have stopped the steroids within 2 years.

FIBROMYALGIA

What abnormalities would you expect on her immunology screen?

You would expect it to be normal. There is the chance however that there may be a positive result, which would give you a dilemma as to whether it is clinically significant.

How likely is she to have joint swelling?

She is very likely to complain that her joints 'feel' swollen, but it would be unlikely for you to see any objective evidence of this swelling.

She asks about a course of steroids. What would you advise?

There is no evidence to support the use of steroids in fibromyalgia. You would explain this to her and also tell her about the potential side effects of steroids.

VASCULITIS

A 41 year old man with asthma, eosinophilia and mononeuritis multiplex.

Churg-Strauss syndrome.

A 41 year old man with chronic sinusitis and a saddle shaped nose.

Wegener's granulomatosis.

A 29 year old IV drug user who is hepatitis C positive.

Cryoglobulinaemia.

A 21 year old Japanese lady with a significant blood pressure difference between her arms.

Takayasu arteritis.

A 41 year old man with a positive p-ANCA, hepatitis B and microaneurysms in the small and medium sized arteries of his kidneys .

Polyarteritis nodosa.

A 9 year old girl with joint pains and a purpuric rash mainly over her buttocks.

Henoch-Schönlein purpura.

A 77 year old man with scalp tenderness and myalgia around his shoulders and hips.

Giant cell arteritis (with associated polymyalgia rheumatica)

A 1 year old boy with inflammation of his lips and tongue and bilateral conjunctivitis.

Kawasaki disease.

What are the two most important management steps?

High dose (60mg) of prednisolone and an ophthalmology review the same day.

In temporal arteritis what should you be able to feel when you palpate for a temporal artery pulse?

No pulse (classically there are tender, enlarged, non-pulsatile temporal arteries).

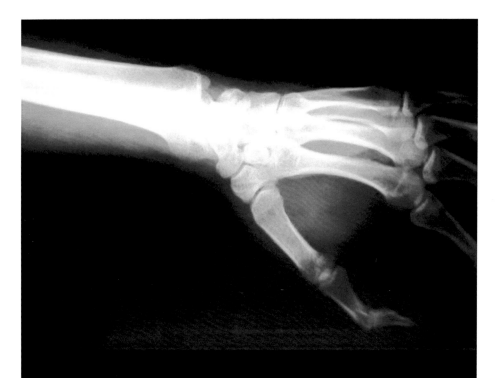

RHEUMATOLOGY

BEST OF FIVE
QUESTIONS

Dr Matthew Langtree

LESS TIME, MORE KNOWLEDGE